LOW LEVEL LASER THERAPY FOR PHYSICAL THERAPISTS

By MALINI CHAUDHRI. Ph.D, L.Ac (WHO. China). ISTE
Edited by JAN TUNER, DDS. SWEDEN

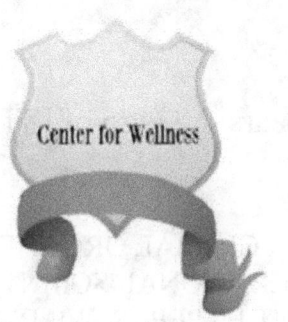

Center for Wellness

CENTER FOR WELLNESS. ISTE
A START UP DEDICATED TO DIGITAL EDUCATION IN
INTEGRATED THERAPIES
IAO VERIFIED IN 2014

CENTER FOR WELLNESS IS LOCATED IN NEW DELHI
OFFICE: D 2 KALINDI. RING ROAD. DELHI 110065. INDIA
IT IS MANAGED AND OWNED BY MALINI CHAUDHRI.

Authors page : http://amazon.com/author/malinichaudhri

Facebook page: https://www.facebook.com/centerforwellness.delhi

Twitter: https://www.twitter.com/maliniwellness

Email: malini@bitrix24.com

All content and certificate bears the logo of ISTE, through kind permissions
granted as LM 71879(2010).

CENTER FOR WELLNESS IS A GLOBAL ORGANIZATION AND INVITES
COLLABORATION WITH EXCEPTIONAL SCIENTISTS, THERAPISTS AND SPA
OR COMPANY MANAGEMENT EXPERTS. WE EMBRACE CHANGE AND
DIGITIZATION AND DEVELOP OUT SYSTEMS IN THE ECOSYSTEM.

Low Level Laser Therapy for Physical Therapists, Second Edition

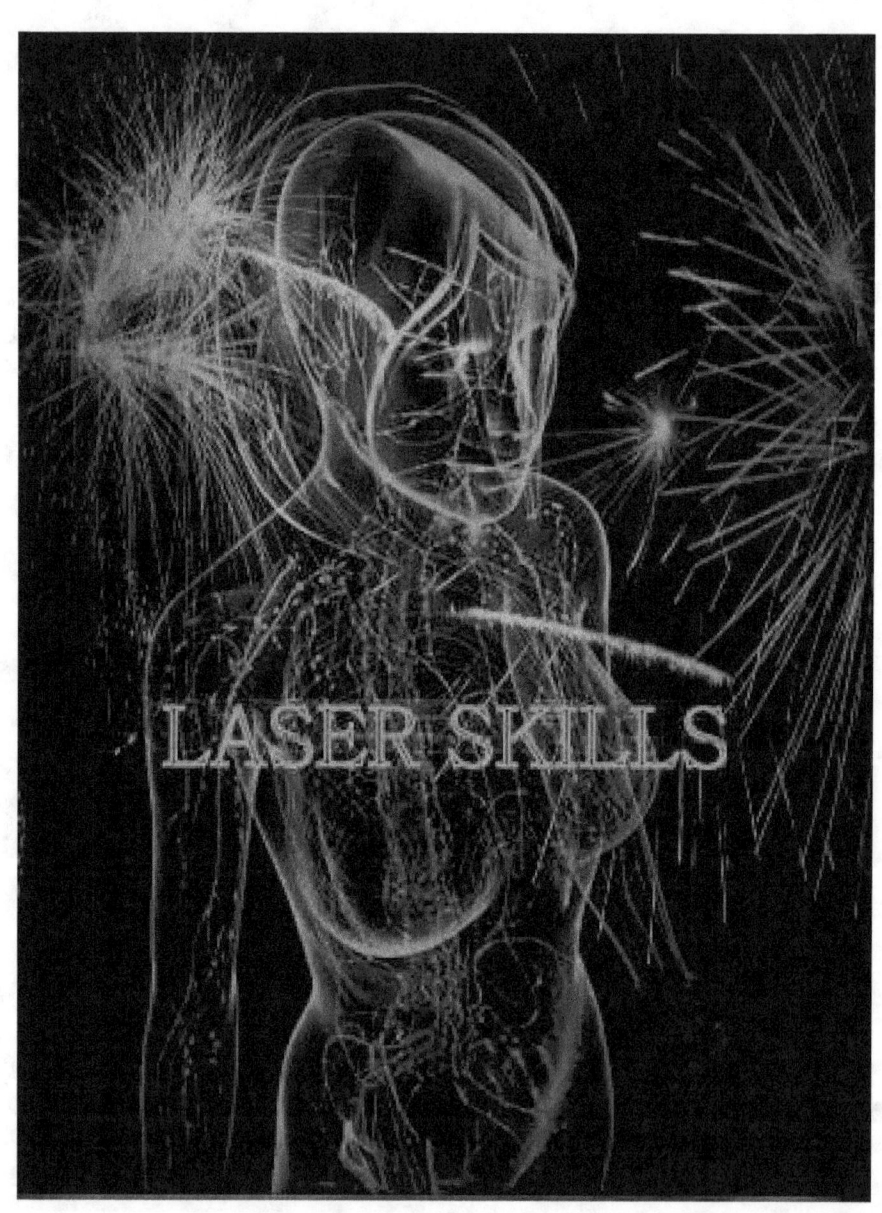

SKILLS DEVELOPMENT IN LOW LEVEL LASER APPLICATIONS FOR OPTIMUM AND PAINLESS RECOVERY

This manual is developed towards a practical online course for physiotherapists and doctors seeking to enhance their skills.

The course manages supplements, guidelines for portfolio of practical's, and assessments on the first five sections.

The science is very vast in its discovery and potential. This manual is restricted to technical structures of application in relation to manual therapies, physical therapy, cam or medi-spa, and has rich sources of evidence which will support all medical practitioners.

The sections reveal interesting approaches to integrated therapy with laser that enhances effects and reduces recovery downtime.

Most interesting is that low level laser heals the DNA, which has great potential in gene support and many new possibilities for healing.

ABOUT THE AUTHOR

Malini Chaudhri was born in Calcutta, India, in 1963. She attended university in Mumbai, and then travelled in 1987 to China where she settled as a Foreign Expert in South China Normal University to teach English to Undergraduates. By 1989 she was promoted to the English Graduate department in the University.

She developed an interest in Chinese medicine, especially laser acupuncture, which was a new modality in 1990. She interacted with experts over seminars in Hong Kong, Taiwan and China.

In 1994, back in Delhi, she was laser consultant to the National Hockey team and Sports Authority of India. Hinduja Sports Foundation awarded her a meritorious grant to cover her Ph.D. fees in Alma Ata University in Sri Lanka. In 2002 she was given a W.H.O (China) International license by Alma Ata which permitted her to practice traditional acupuncture outside of China.

The Low Level Laser Therapy system was fast emerging as a specialized science. Laser acupuncture was far from understood. The author met with the leading team of laser scientists in Chennai at the ISLSM meet. In 2002 She travelled to Tsukuba to attend the 4th WALT World Congress and presented a trial on National Women's golf. An editorial appeared in Laser World which showed laser acupuncture as a modality that could give relief to golfers during times of harsh weather. Premsyl Fryda published two scientific papers authored by Malini Chaudhri in Laser Partner Journal, published by the Czech Republic.

In 2003 she was invited through personal sponsorship to the U.S. She attended the NAALT Congress at Bethesda and attended professional development courses in the US in Lymphology, Sports massage and Medical Acupuncture.

After 2004 the author was actively involved with application in sports as horse Polo, and golf. She was consultant to many celebrated international sports persons. For some time she assisted a neurosurgeon with laser. The Spa industry came up by 2007, and the author took a lead role in developing world class spas in Heritage hotels and Indian Palaces of living monarchs. In 2008 she managed the verification of the Habia qualification in India which was successfully verified by the UK team. Soon after she became a life member of Indian Society of Technical Education, and developed the Center for Wellness as a Skills Knowledge Provider in the wellness industry, based on MOU. She integrated with CAM sector in hospitals and provided research on orthopaedic management, tendonitis and stroke rehabilitation. She managed CME seminars for hospitals which was appreciated.

WITH KIND COURTESY VALUABLE EDITORIAL CONTRIBUTIONS ARE FROM JAN TUNÉR

A vote of thanks to Jan Tunér for his support, time, and rich knowledge in this subject which has been shared with me in full LLLT has emerged during the past two decades with infinite possibilities. Jan Tuner has made a lot of this possible by establishing the scientific doctrine through his book, co-authored with Lars Hode, through his appointments as newsletter editor and Secretary General of WALT, and through his editorial management of Laser World, and his activities with Swedish Medical Laser Society.

Jan Tunér has supported India with his book donated to me for the development of laser knowledge in India and remained consistently, a profound scientific mentor to me and the laser scientist fraternity. In this course, we are proud recipients of his grace and editorial advice which has upgraded out text into a new generation model of knowledge awareness. LLLT may possibly become the future of medicine.

Publications by Jan Tunér, DDS. Detailed reference to meritorious scientific publications are listed at the end of the manual.
Jan Tunér: General Manager, Prima Books AB, Sweden. President, Dala Dental. Sweden.

Publications : BOOKS
Tunér J, Hode L. Dental laser be handling. 1992. Svenska Laser-Medicinska Sällskapet, Stockholm.
Tunér J, Hode L. Lågeffekts laser i odontologin. 1995. Svenska Laser-Medicinska Sällskapet.
TunérJ, Hode L. Laser Therapy in Dentistry and Medicine. 1996. Prima Books, Sweden.
Tunér J, Hode L, Diklic S. Laser u Stomatologiji. 1996. Novi Sad, Yugoslavia.
Tunér J, Hode L. Low Level Laser Therapy, clinical practice and scientific background. 1999. Prima Books, Sweden.
Tunér J, Hode L. Laser therapy, clinical practice and scientific background. 2002. Prima Books, Sweden.
Tunér J, Hode L. The Laser Therapy Handbook. Prima Books,Sweden, 2004.
Tunér J, Hode L. Laser therapy, clinical practice and scientific background. Korean translation. 2006.
Tunér J, Hode L. Laser therapy, clinical practice and scientific background. Greek translation. 2008.
Tunér J, Hode L. The New Laser Therapy Handbook. 2010. Prima Books, Sweden.
Jan Tunér, Per Hugo Kristensen. Low Level Lasers in Dentistry. In: Convissar B (ed).

Editorial positions:
Editorial board member of the Journal "Laser Therapy" 1996-2001.
Editorial board member of "Photo medicine and Laser Surgery" 2002 - Present
Editor in chief, WALT Review 2000 – Present
Editorial board member, The Internet Journal of Laser needle Medicine 2006 – present

Reviewer of Photo medicine and Laser Surgery
Reviewer of Lasers in Medical Science
Reviewer of Angle Orthodontics
Reviewer of Lasers in Surgery and Medicine
Reviewer of Current Rheumatology
Reviewer of Journal of Photochemistry & Photobiology B: Biology
Reviewer Medical Science Monitor 2010Senior editor of Laser, International magazine of Laser Dentistry 2009 – present

Continued at back of book

AUTHORIZED AND REGULATED BY INDIAN SOCIETY OF TECHNICAL EDUCATION.

India's premier, most honoured technical board has reviewed the competency and credentials of the author, and accepted her to develop skills, vocational courses for institutions and wellness centres

This certificate course bears its logo for authenticity and quality.
We are proud recipients of their mandate.
Special thanks to Dr. Professor Ranjit Singh, former Secretary, ISTE and Editor of ISTE Journal.

ISTE LM NO 71879(2010)

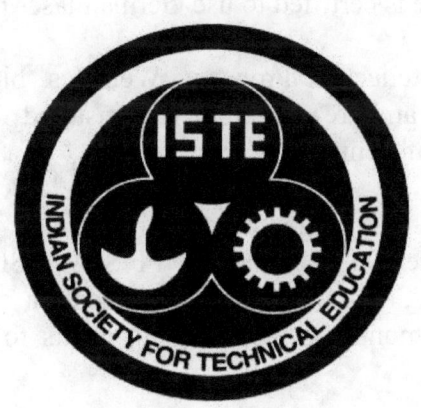

QUALITY ASSURED

The Centre for Wellness was assessed for accreditation by IAO, USA, in May 2014, and was approved as successful Candidate for accreditation. The site and technical data of this course and company was externally verified. The Company structure and merit listing of authors, editors, and advisors was also evaluated and marked successful.

ISTE (under societies registration act xxi of 1860) has issued Malini Chaudhri Life Membership and IP no **LM 71879 (2010),** MOU (Judicial) M273667.
Center for Wellness. Registration under Companies Act 1908, enrollment no D/640/2009 on 29/9.2010.
Dr. Ac International license in conformity with the W.H.O syllabus of 1974. Issued from Beijing. License No Ac 12.02.211 4C.

The author is associated with many Laser Scientific groups as ISLA, WALT, NAALT, ISLMS and EMLA. A senior member of EMLA has awarded her certificates of merit based on journal IP no ISSN 1213-3027, 1213-1156, the Journal being named Laser Partner from Czech Republic.

The author is US licensed in Sports massage, Lymphatic Drainage therapy, and Medical Acupuncture of Nogier. She is certified to use German laser physio of Weberneedles.

All content is protected Intellectual Property. Websites, blogs and domains, business email bear SSL certificates and are copyrighted, registered for international trade mark, and owned by the Founder of Center for Wellness.

The content is also based on privileged community support from a medical community hospital bearing the license No.BH/PERS-IV/PF/SEWA/301/2011. This hospital has provided the certificate for Continuing Medical Education of Low level Laser therapy. This non-profit based community is also bearing rights to the IP and copyrights for archiving purposes.

CONTENTS

Interspersed with editorial updates

Continued profile of Jan Tuner

PREFACE TO THE SECTIONS

This manual is for Skills development in therapists needing to upgrade from manual therapy to low level laser therapy. It will support practical training in fitness therapists, physical therapists, CAM therapists and advanced spa therapists. It will also support patients who need to know or asses their therapist's skills in order to achieve the most of their treatment regimen.

LLLT does not come with cook book formulas, so be receptive to the experience of the particular therapist.

The first section is an introduction to LLLT with precise support to its basic background and development in clinical practise. Jan Tuner has offered valuable inputs on the directions of the new treatment modality in its scope for reversing serious disease or managing conditions.

The second section discusses many aspects of safety in practise. This is so that mistakes can be circumvented that cause the business, laser or scientific arena to be mistrusted.

The third section is applicable to the muscle anatomy and approaches to accelerate healing time. The techniques come under myofascial dysfunction.

The fourth section is based on lymphatic drainage and reconstruction and the impact of the science on managing lymphedema, cancer prevention and post-surgical clinical support.

The fifth section is based on laser acupuncture and frequencies used for various concerns that are mental, psychological, and emotional or even limbic (primitive). Micro acupuncture is also discussed which is known for de-addiction, weight loss, metabolic syndrome, sedation, anaesthesia and similar.

The final session reviews recent clinical data on intravenous laser, which treats systemic diseases based on blood and circulatory problems.

SECTION ONE

LLLT IN SKILLS DEVELOPMENT

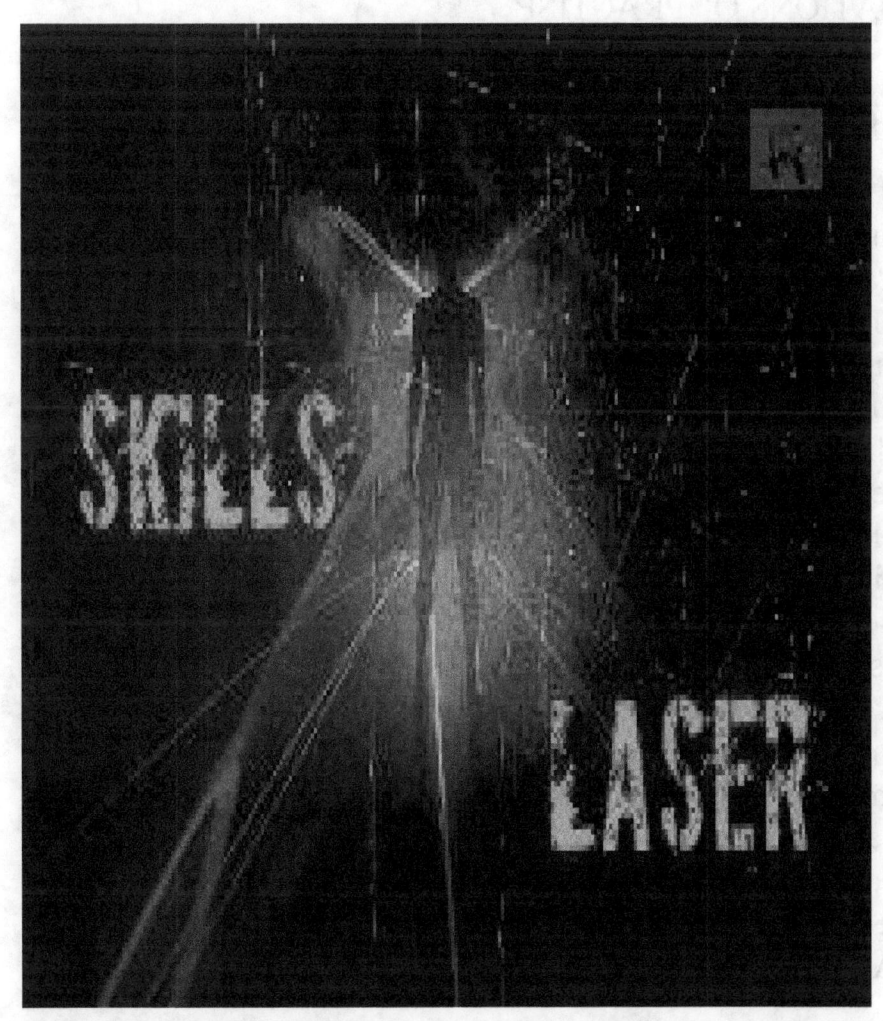

LASERS IN SCIENTIFIC PRACTISE
THE NATURE OF LOW LEVEL LASER THERAPY IN HEALING
PRACTICAL KNOWLEDGE

SKILLS DEVELOPMENT IN THIS SECTION

KNOWLEDGE OF LASER SPECIFICATIONS AND MECHANISMS
PRINCIPLES OF APPLICATION
WALT DOSE RECOMMENDATIONS
EDITORIAL CONTRIBUTIONS. New generation laser therapy
FOUNDATIONS OF PRACTISE

CONTENTS

KNOW YOUR LASER : COMMON PARAMETERS

Helium Neon 630-685 nm, In Ga AIP red laser light
780 – 830 nm, Ga AlAs slightly visible red laser light
904 nm, Ga As super pulsed. Invisible laser light
10.600 nm.CO2 laser. Invisible light

When using a therapeutic laser in vivo, we need to consider many additional parameters. If most of the laser light is absorbed in the dermis, for example, then we cannot achieve an optimal effect. When laser light hits tissue, it can be absorbed, scattered (including reflection), or transmitted. The main components in tissue that we need to consider are: melanin, oxyhaemoglobin, deoxyhemoglobin, and water. We can get light into the body with wavelengths from 600 nm (red end of the spectrum) to 1100 nm (near infrared end of the spectrum). The range is often referred to as the "therapeutic window" for laser applications.

Although these wavelengths can penetrate, each wavelength has unique penetration characteristics. If we put an ordinary white light source, a flashlight, into the palm of our hand, we will see a red glow out the other side. Longer wavelengths such as red penetrate deeper.
The amount of red light visibly seen through the hand is dependent on the colour of the skin. Melanin absorbs light strongly, so dark skin will absorb more light, especially wavelengths from 500 nm to 800 nm. Wavelengths longer than 1200 nm absorb in water very strongly and therefore it is difficult to get much penetration in tissue. These longer wavelength lasers are typically used in ablative procedures such as surgery or skin resurfacing.

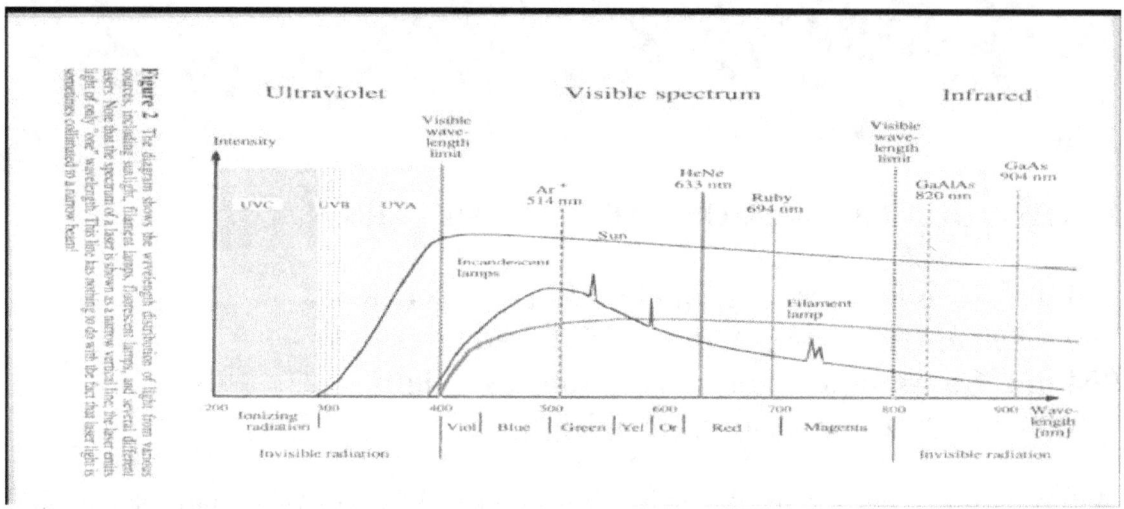

Courtesy Jan Tuner.

ACTION SPECTRUM

Editorial selection on recent literature

Karu recalls the basic LAWS OF PHOTOCHEMISTRY
The first law of photochemistry (Grotthus-Draper Law) states that a molecule before photochemistry must absorb light. LLLT is concerned with the photo acceptor.

The second law of photochemistry (Stark-Einstein law) states that light absorbed need not necessarily result in photochemistry, but if it does, only one photon is required for each affected molecule. This indicates a relatively short life span of an electronically excited molecule and the relatively low concentration of incident photons in most conventional systems.
Photons carry a level of energy that depend on their wavelength and this wavelength can be transferred into a molecular entity by absorption.
The absorption spectrum is the spectrum of radiant energy whose intensity at each wavelengths a measure of the amount of the amount of energy at that wavelength that has passed through a selectively absorbing substance.
The action spectrum, means the efficiency with which electromagnetic radiation produces a photochemical reaction.

ACTION SPECTRA

The radiation wavelengths effective for photobiology range between 300 and 900 nm, i.e., from UV (ultraviolet) to near IR (infrared). Practically all photo biological processes in plants and animals, such as photosynthesis,

16

phototropism, photo taxis, photo periodism, and vision, utilize this range of radiation. The photoreceptor molecules responsible for these photo responses have well studied for decades.

The regulation of cellular metabolism by visible light is not a classical topic of photobiology.

Only the finding of the existence of action spectra in the region from 330 to 860 nm for the increase of DNA and RNA synthesis rates in mammalian cells, as well as for growth stimulation of eukaryotic and prokaryotic microorganisms recorded in the 1980's, indicated that monochromatic light in the visible-to-near visible region can be a subtle instrument to regulate cellular metabolism. This finding means that the topic of low level laser phototherapy. (or low level light therapy, or laser bio stimulation) belongs to photobiology.

An action spectrum is a plot of the relative effectiveness of different wavelengths of light in causing a particular biological response, and under ideal conditions, it should mimic the absorption spectrum of the molecule that is absorbing the light, and whose photochemical alteration causes the effect.

The action spectra in the visible-to-near IR region for the biological responses of cultured cells showed that red light at 632.8 nm was not the only wavelength suitable for laser bio stimulation.

These spectra together with the results of experiments using the dichromatic irradiation of cells, and the modification of light effects with chemicals, showed that "laser bio stimulation" is a photo biological phenomenon. These data also allowed the suggestion that the photo acceptor for the stimulation of cell metabolism is the terminal enzyme of the respiratory chain, i.e., cytochrome c oxidase for eukaryotic cells, and the cytochrome complex for Escherichia coli.

In the blue spectral region, flavo proteins like NADH-dehydrogenase can work as photo acceptors as well. The suggestion that cytochrome c oxidase is the photo acceptor molecule has been recently confirmed in elegant experiments with functionally inactivated primary neurons, proposing that light up regulates this enzyme.

2. ACTION SPECTRA for an INCREASE of DNA and RNA SYNTHESIS RATE in CULTURED MAMMALIAN CELLS

First at all, let us remember that in eukaryotic cells, DNA and RNA synthesis occur in the nucleus, which does not have chromophores absorbing in the spectral region used for laser phototherapy (600-900 nm).

the wavelength range used in our experiments, and important for phototherapy (600-860 nm), there are four "active" regions, but the peak positions are not exactly the same for all action spectra. The red band has a peak position between 613.5 and 623.5 nm (in one spectrum, at 606 nm); the far-red band has peak positions between 667.5 and 683.7 nm, and two near IR bands in the range of 750.7-772.3 nm and 812.5-846.0 nm.

3. INTERPRETATION of the ACTION SPECTRA: CYTOCHROME C OXIDASE is the PHOTOACCEPTOR MOLECULE

In the beginning of the 90's, the earlier action spectra were analysed using all available spectroscopic literature data which allowed forming a suggestion about the chromophores involved. Bear in mind that the chromophores are the components of molecules that absorb the light.

A number of other kinds of experiments (dose and intensity dependences for various wavelengths, dichromatic irradiation in various ways modification of irradiation experiments by specific chemicals, and others) were performed. The results of all these experiments, together with action spectroscopy experiments, allowed the conclusion that cytochrome c oxidase could be a universal photo acceptor for eukaryotic cells.

4. COMPARISON of ACTION and ABSORPTION SPECTRA

Insofar as an action spectrum mirrors the absorption spectrum of the molecule that absorbs the light and is responsible for the action spectrum recorded, an important step in identification of this photo absorbing molecule is the comparison of action and absorption spectra.
The comparison of action spectra connected with reactions in the cellular nucleus, and the absorption spectra of cellular monolayers at 600-860 nm allow one to conclude that by peak positions, these two groups of spectra may belong to the same molecule.

5. MITOCHONDRIAL SIGNALING: HOW the LIGHT-GENERATED SIGNAL in MITOCHONDRIA can INFLUENCE CELLULAR METABOLISM

We know from the action spectra that the DNA and RNA synthesis rate is influenced by irradiation, and we know that the photo acceptor (tentatively cytochrome c oxidase) is located in mitochondria. There is an important question left: how the signal generated by the light quanta in cytochrome c oxidase is transduced to the nucleus. The answer is that mitochondrial retrograde signalling quite probable is responsible for this.

Recent work has uncovered an impressive number of extra mitochondrial factors that regulate the expression of nuclear genes for mitochondrial proteins. However, relatively little is known about how mitochondria send signals to the nucleus, and how the nucleus controls the expression of individual genes. One pathway of communication in cells from mitochondria to the nucleus that influences many cellular activities under both normal and pathophysiological conditions is mitochondrial retrograde signalling. This recently discovered signalling is an opposite signalling pathway to a common and well defined pathway transforming information from the nucleus and cytoplasm to the mitochondria. Mitochondrial retrograde signalling sends information back to the nucleus about changes in the functional state of the mitochondria.

The existence of a cellular signalling pathway: mitochondria cytoplasm (plasma membrane cytoplasm) nucleus, was proposed in 1988 . The reason to suggest the existence of such a cellular signalling pathway (then named photo signal transduction and amplification chain) was simple. It appeared that the action spectra for the increase of DNA and RNA synthesis rate could be recorded when cultured cells are irradiated in the region From 300 to 860 nm. The nucleus does not have chromospheres absorbing in this region.

Secondly, the data gathered to date showed that photo acceptors are located in the respiratory chain. So, it was then logical to suppose the existence of cellular signalling cascades between organelles. In 2004, a novel mitochondrial-signalling pathway in mammalian cells activated by red and near IR radiation was discovered. It was shown by Schroeder et al that IR-A radiation (760-1440 nm), in contrast to UV radiation, elicits a retrograde signalling response in normal human skin fibroblasts.

Fig. 1.3

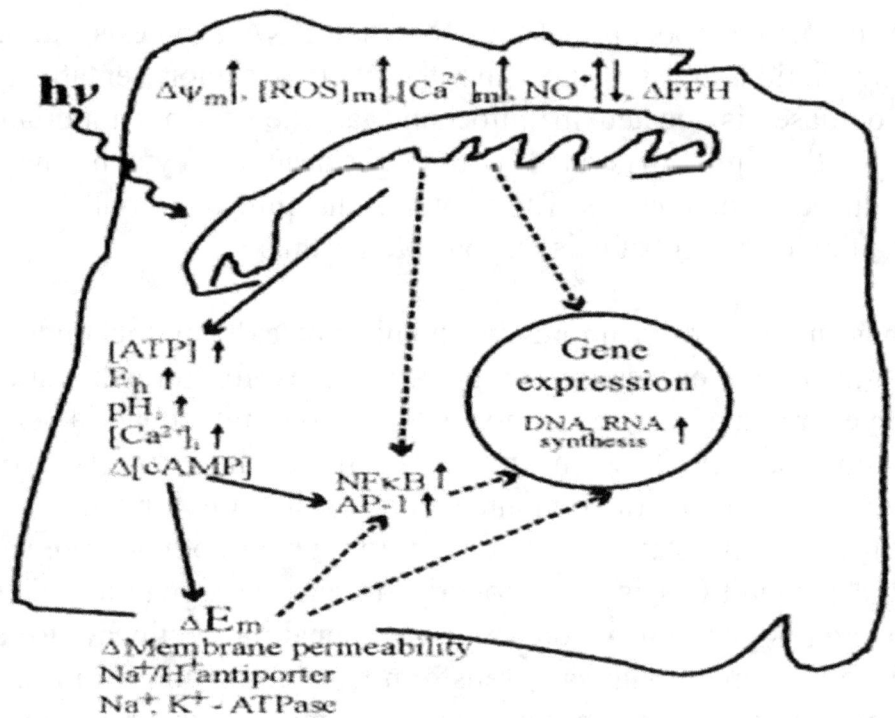

There is every reason to believe, on the basis of experimental data gathered so far, that mitochondrial retrograde signalling, a recently discovered cellular signalling pathway, functions also in irradiated cells.

Modulation of retrograde mitochondrial signalling elements like , $(ROS)m$, $(Ca2+)m$ in irradiated cells is rather well documented (review: 73). Also, the responses to irradiation occurring in the nucleus (i.e., increase in DNA and RNA synthesis rate, and expression of genes of various function categories) are definitely documented. However, the pathways of light signal transduction between these two ends needs further investigation.

SUMMARY

1. The similarity of action spectra for different cellular responses suggests that the photo acceptor is the same for these responses. For the responses reported here, the photo acceptor appears to be cytochrome c oxidase. Recall that it was suggested in 1981 that photosensitivity might be a common mitochondrial property in higher animals, and could have physiological significance under certain conditions, e.g., exposure to orange-red light, and high ADP levels.

2. Based on these action spectra, various wavelengths can be used for low level light therapy, *i.e. those around 404, 620, 680, 760, and 820 nm.*

3. The existence of the action spectra for biochemical processes occurring in various cellular organelles (nucleus, plasma membrane) assume the existence of cellular signalling pathways between a photo acceptor in the mitochondria and the nucleus, as well as between photo acceptor and the plasma membrane.

4. It is believed that the "mitochondrial mechanism" of low level light therapy works in all types of cells containing mitochondria.

Recent literature on LLLT is based on the exciting possibilities of the mitochondria, under laser irradiation, to induce healing of a very advanced nature. Learners must acknowledge the giant leap forward that laser medicine is undergoing. Our course exists in a classical framework of fundamentals.

1.1 IN PRACTISE - LASER TREATMENT MODES

Having understood the laser and the scientific background, the next step is to focus on modes of practical application.

Laser treatments are classified under the systems listed below, in relation to anatomical, local and general effects. Skills in each mode has to be achieved

Tissue and wound repair

Lymphtic drainage

Trigger point therapy

Acupuncture.
Auriculotherapy

Pain Management

1.2 LASER THERAPY TECHNIQUES

Below are practical steps to achieve precise results.
Wavelength, spot size, power and
Other factors must be consider

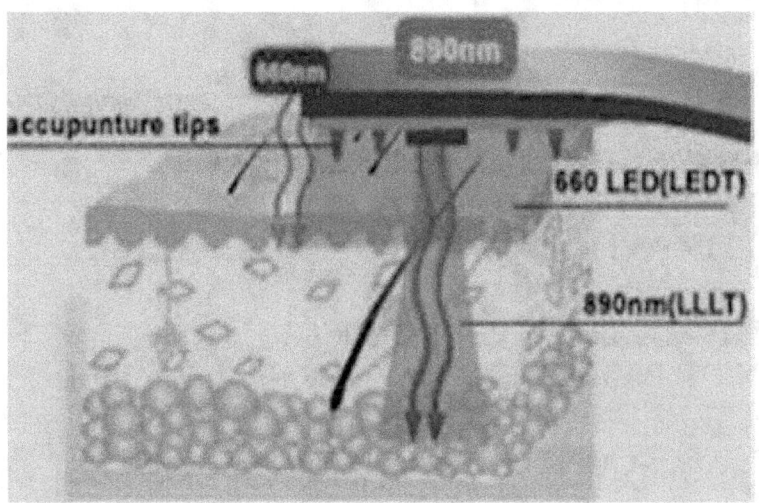

PROXIMAL PRIORITY. OSHIRO'S PRINCIPLE

Prioritize treatment of pathological tissue (consider oedema, pain swelling, wound or other in designing dose and treatment protocol).

PRESSURE:

WOODPECKER TECHNIQUE : *(*Apply pressure, release, again apply pressure).

ISCHEMIC PRESSURE : Apply deep stationary pressure on trigger points/acupuncture points in contact mode

---

SCANNING
For large areas. Maybe in stationary
mode or scanning in close proximity to skin

INTRAVENOUS laser, which penetrates into the vein and passes laser through the blood.

1.3 DOSAGE

Assess the factors listed below to arrive at your dose parameters.

-LASER WAVELENGTH (DEGREE OF PENETRATION)
-LASER POWER OUTPUT (POWER DENSITY)
-SKIN PHOTO TYPE (FITZPATRICK). TYPE 4-6 ARE DARK SKINS, 1-3 ARE FAIR.
-TYPE OF TISSUE (OEDEMA TIC, FATTY, MUSCULAR)
DEPTH OF LOCATION OF PATHOLOGY. SUPERFICIAL TISSUE VS. DEEP TISSUE
-MODE OF CONTACT: NON-CONTACT/CONTACT/ FIRM CONTACT/ PRESSURE
-CONTACT
-ACUTE/CHRONIC CONDITION
-DIAGNOSTIC SKILLS
-KNOWLEDGE SKILL OF THERAPIST

DOSES ARE CUMMULATIVE. Daily doses as per recommendations are more effective than the entire dose in a single session, except in the application of Pontinen's Principle in Physical Therapy.

EDITORIAL MESSAGE Important parameters
From Tunér-Hode

A)Wavelength

That biological effect is
significantly related
to the wavelength of the light emitted
by the laser has been demonstrated
in numerous studies. Today, the wavelengths most
commonly used for therapeutic purposes are
633 nm (HeNe lasers), 635 nm, 650 nm, 660
nm, 670 nm (In GaAIP lasers), 780 nm, 820
nm, 830 nm (GaAIAs lasers), 904 nm
(GaAs lasers), and 10600 nm (CO2 lasers).
Except for GaAs and CO2 lasers, all these
lasers usually produce a continuous beam
but may also be pulsed.

B) Dose

The most important parameter in LLLT is always the dose, often referred to as "fluence". By dose (D) is meant the energy (E) of the light directed at a given unit of area (A) during a given session of therapy. The energy is measured in J (joules), the area in cm2, and, consequently, the dose in J/cm2. Mathematically, this may be expressed as follows:

$$D = \frac{E}{A} \quad [J/cm2]$$

Assuming that the power (P) output of the laser probe remains constant during treatment, the energy (E) of the light will be equal to the power multiplied by the time (t) during which the light is emitted. The dose may then be calculated as follows:

$$D = \frac{P\,t}{A} \quad [J/cm2]$$

Sometimes, however, the power output is not constant, such as when the laser is pulsed or modulated, which may be achieved in several ways. The preferred method of pulsing a HeNe laser is to use some form of mechanical switching device or shutter, such as a rotating pierced disc, the useful proportion of the time during which light is emitted by the laser normally being fixed at a given value (duty cycle), most often 50%. In other words, light is permitted to pass through the disc for 50% of the total operating time (and is blocked for the remaining 50%). This enables use of the concepts of mean power (Pm) and maximum power. In the example given here, the mean power is 50% of the maximum power. If the laser is pulsed at mean power, the above formula will apply, giving:

$$D = \frac{P_m \, t}{A} \quad [J/cm2]$$

GA As lasers always pulse, the duration of each pulse being extremely short, and in these lasers the maximum power is always much, much greater than the mean power. This type of pulsing is often referred to as super-pulsing. In GA As lasers, the duration of the pulse is normally in the region of 100-200 ns (nanoseconds) and the maximum power is typically 1 - 20 W (watts). Assuming, for example, that the duration of the pulse is 150 ns and that the maximum power is 10 W, each pulse emitted by the laser will have an energy of 1.5 µ J (micro joules).

If the laser emits 100 such pulses per second (a pulse frequency of 100 Hz), its mean power output will be 0.15 mw (mill watts). A pulse frequency of 1000 Hz gives a mean output of 1.5 mw, etc. In other words, the mean power output varies with the number of pulses emitted per second. By applying these relationships, it is often possible to obtain doses or other parameters not explicitly stated in the article under review.

C) Power density
Power density, indicating the degree of concentration of the power output, has also increasingly proved to play a major role. It is measured in watts per square centimetre (W/cm2). If, for example, a circular area having a diameter of 5 mm (approx. 0.2

cm2) is illuminated with a laser operating at a power output of 100 mw, the biological effects are quite different from those produced by illuminating a circular area of 5 cm diameter (approx. 20 cm2) with the same laser. In the first case, the power density is 100 times greater than the second. Some studies have concluded that the power density may be of even greater significance than the dose. This parameter is very seldom indicated in the articles we have studied. It must also be remembered that the power density varies within the area illuminated - normally, it will be greatest at the centre.

1.4 CONTRAINDICATIONS

Do not attempt to use laser therapy in the following conditions:
*Cancer/malignancy
*Pregnancy
*Thyroid (direct exposure over glands)
*Direct exposure to the eye
*The PT should use LLLT in conjunction with drugs if necessary
*And manage cases comprehensively.
*LLLT practitioners should not claim outcomes

1.5 MECHANISMS OF ACTION OF LASER LIGHT

Diffuse or targeted scattering of laser light in tissue gives interference and speckle formation.

Primary mechanisms:
1. Volumes of partially polarized light are formed

The absorption of polarized light in cytochrome molecules (e.g. Porphyries), stimulates the creation of singlet oxygen and ATPase.

2. Points of high laser intensity appear
In points of high intensity the probability of multi photon effects is higher. The electrical field across the cell membrane creates a dipole moment on the bar shaped lipids.

3. Areas of high difference in light intensity levels form
Local differences in intensity create temperature and pressure gradients across cell membranes.

Secondary mechanisms:
PROMOTE WOUND HEALING
The laser wavelength and intensity produces an increase of ATP ase and activation of CAMP and enzymes.
This triggers an immunological chain reaction which activates macrophages – increases mast cells- and enhances S.R.F to precipitate wound healing. It increases procollagen synthesis in fibroblasts –thereby increasing endothelial cells and keratinocytes which influences wound healing.

INFLUENCE ON INFLAMMATION

Points of high intensity laser, and areas with different levels of light intensity, experience a reaction in the permeability of cell membrane. This has effect on the Ca2+, Na+ and K+ as well as the proton gradient over the mitochondria membranes.
This phenomenon influences inflammation by increasing serotonin level in the blood, and by enhancing the S.O.D levels.

INFLUENCE ON PAIN

The primary mechanisms effects on cell membrane permeability cause a further reaction seen as increased receptor activity of cell membranes. There is an enhanced synthesis of endorphins, a decrease of Bradykinin, a decrease of c-fibre activity, and increased nerve cell action potential.
Action of low level laser induced photo bio modulation in target tissues is shown in the chart below.

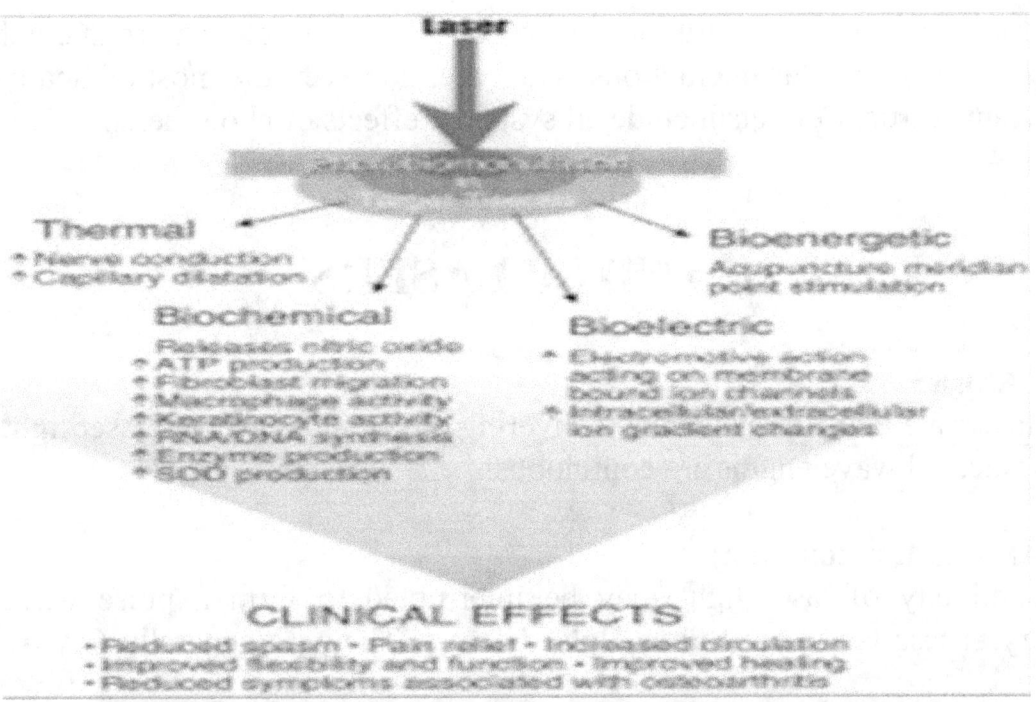

Laser

Thermal
* Nerve conduction
* Capillary dilatation

Bioenergetic
Acupuncture meridian point stimulation

Biochemical
* Releases nitric oxide
* ATP production
* Fibroblast migration
* Macrophage activity
* Keratinocyte activity
* RNA/DNA synthesis
* Enzyme production
* SOD production

Bioelectric
* Electromotive action acting on membrane bound ion channels
* Intracellular/extracellular ion gradient changes

CLINICAL EFFECTS
* Reduced spasm * Pain relief * Increased circulation
* Improved flexibility and function * Improved healing
* Reduced symptoms associated with osteoarthritis

1.6 MORE ON MECHANISMS OF PHOTO THERAPY

Mary Dyson has classified phototherapy and its effects on the body into primary, secondary and tertiary effects. It is the unique synergy between the three responses that create the phototherapeutic effect. The primary effects are created by direct photoreception of photons with cytochromes resulting in increases in ATP production and changes in cell membrane permeability; this response is specific to phototherapy. Photoreception is generally followed by transduction of light into cellular energy, amplification of the signal and a photo response, the last of which can be classified as either secondary or tertiary.

Secondary effects occur in the same cell in which photons produced the primary effects; they are induced by these primary effects. Secondary effects include cell proliferation, protein synthesis, degranulation, growth factor secretion myofibroblast contraction and neurotransmitter modification, depending on the cell type and its sensitivity. They are less predictable than primary effects; the sensitivity of the cells is dependent on internal and external environment factors.

The tertiary effects are the indirect responses of distant cells to changes in other cells that have interacted directly with photons. They are the least predictable because they are dependent on both variable environmental factors and intercellular interactions. They are, however, the most clinically significant. Tertiary effects include all systemic effects of phototherapy.

1.7 CW LASERS AND SP LASERS

CW LASERS
Most lasers are **Continuous wave**, delivering direct, uninterrupted laser light Into tissue. All wavelengths are continuous.

SP LASERS(less common)
The continuity of laser light may be interrupted to form a pulse wave delivery. These lasers are **Super Pulsed** lasers. They are generally GA As lasers.
SP lasers have a lower average intensity and a single pulse of a much higher Intensity that drives photons into deeper tissue. An SP laser might have a delivery of 15 mw average interrupted by a single pulse output of 50 Watts.
A third kind of laser has a chopped pulsing. It is a crude mechanism of on/off of the laser beam. This laser is the least preferred in laser therapy practice.

Lasers come in popular DIY commercial models as laser combs laser apparatus for full body in baths and beds and even IR rooms. These have timed protocols and SOPS and induce generalized healing or photon stimulation. These apparatus must not be confused with the targeted clinical applications applied in this manual.

INTRAVENOUS LASERS
These lasers are recent inventions for blood irradiation and anti-cancer treatment. They are used for systemic diseases based on circulatory problems. The fibre tips penetrate the vein and the laser in 5 mw or less strength, red, blue or green wavelengths, and activate blood purification and energy mechanisms deep within the body.

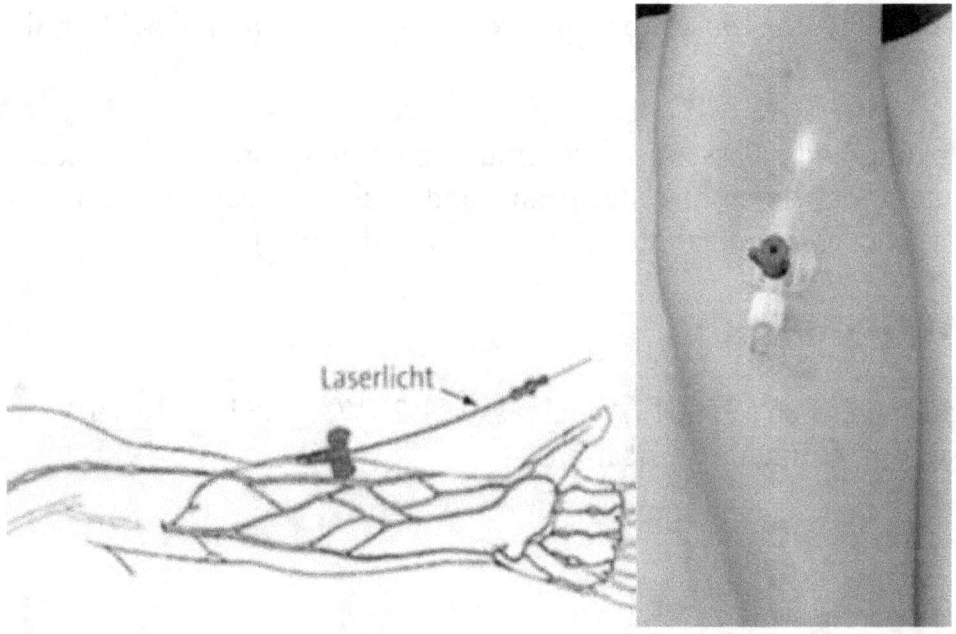

Laserlicht

Image taken from the International Journal ISLA edition. Weber needle technology

1.8 PONTINEN'S PRINCIPLE

Continuous wave (CW) laser requires a dosage in joules to elicit a phototherapeutic response. Pontinen's Principle is designed to maximize treatment response in a single visit and to ensure that sufficient dosage has been provided. The technique is to palpate the spasm and have the patient rate their pain. The laser is used to administer 6-8 J/cm2 directly to the spasm. Upon completion of the treatment, clinicians will reassess for pain response. If pain persists, two additional applications may be given to get a treatment response.

Unlike CW lasers, super pulsed lasers emit beams that are always pulsed to set frequencies.

Generally, higher frequencies are used to stimulate tissue and for the relaxation of muscle spasm. Dosimetry for SP lasers is usually given in unit time (seconds), rather than joules. After assessing the patient's pain and spasticity of the muscle, set a frequency between 700 and 2500 Hz with the

SP laser and apply the dose for approximately 2-3 minutes with mild overpressure.

After re-palpating and re-assessing, continued pain or spasm can be treated up to two additional times to reduce pain and spasm. (Keep in mind that pulsed frequencies recommendations are general indicators).

EDITORIAL INSIGHTS.

Posted by Jan Tunér,Feb 19, 2017Annals Issue 1 2017, <u>Annals of Laser Therapy Research</u>, Clinical Applications

To pulse or not to pulse, that is the question

By Jan Tunér

The question of pulsing therapeutic light is not resolved and still rather controversial. This article is an edited version of a chapter in the 2014 book "Laser Phototherapy – Clinical Practice and Scientific Background" (Prima Books).

<u>Pulsed or continuous light</u>

A laser can work continuously (most typical for InGaAlP, HeNe, and GaAlAs lasers) or pulsed (such as the GaAs laser). The GaAs laser (904 or 905 nm) is always super-pulsed, with two possible consequences. Firstly, the pulsing of the laser light may interfere with other pulsing phenomena in the organism, and secondly, continuous/switched and super-pulsed lasers may have different active depths of penetration. A super-pulsed laser always penetrates deeper than a continuous or switched laser with the same wavelength and the same average output power. The extremely intense light flashes of the GaAs laser achieve greater light intensity extending deeper into the tissue.

<u>Pulse repetition rate (PRR)</u>

Few aspects of laser therapy cause so much confusion as the concept of pulsing. So let us try to make it a bit easier.

1.   It is important to understand the difference between "<u>switching</u>" and "<u>super pulsing</u>". Continuous lasers can be pulsed through mechanical or electronical devices. This means that the continuous beam is shut on and off.

The power of the beam remains the same. If the "on-time" and the "off-time" are the same, then the so called "duty cycle" is 50%. This means that the average laser power is 50% of the continuous wave power. If the laser is in the on mode during 90% of the cycle time, then the duty cycle is 90%, i.e. close to continuous. With 50% duty cycle the treatment time has to be doubled in order to achieve the same [energy or energy density] dose as with a continuous beam.

1.9 PONTINEN'S PRINCIPLE

Continuous wave (CW) laser requires a dosage in joules to elicit a phototherapeutic response. Pontinen's Principle is designed to maximize treatment response in a single visit and to ensure that sufficient dosage has been provided. The technique is:

To palpate the spasm and have the patient rate their pain. The laser is used to administer 6-8 J/cm2 directly to the spasm. Upon completion of the treatment, clinicians will reassess for pain response. If pain persists, two additional applications may be given toget a treatment response
Unlike CW lasers, super pulsed lasers emit beams that are always pulsed to set frequencies.

Generally, higher frequencies are used to stimulate tissue and for the relaxation of muscle spasm. Dosimetry for SP lasers is usually given in unit time (seconds), rather than joules. After assessing the patient's pain and spasticity of the muscle, set a frequency between 700 and 2500 Hz with the SP laser and apply the dose for approximately 2-3 minutes with mild overpressure.

After re-palpating and re-assessing, continued pain or spasm can be treated up to two additional times to reduce pain and spasm. (Keep in mind that pulsed frequencies recommendations are general indicators).

Editorial overview

Recent literature from Karu has reflected that in pulsed laser treatments, the action is significant within the dark area between pulses. In some treatments, the inert moment between pulses can reduce progression of cellular activity that is possible from a continuous wave laser supply.

Pulsed laser radiation with a certain set of parameters produced a statistically significant decrease in the intracellular ATP concentration. This result is different from results received by irradiating with CW light.

Karu: The CW radiation of a laser may be used in pulsed mode by switching on and off, but a true pulsed laser may not work in CW mode.
Tunér: Wavelengths determines treatment depth and tissue response, not pulsing. And pulsed laser energies are difficult to calculate except if the laser itself provides indications.

1.10 LASER SPECKLES

HODE'S PRINCIPLE
Coherent laser light was found to have speckles. This causes interference when applied on tissue indicating points of high impact and points of low impact. This creates a phenomenon in medicine that has to be understood by the Physical Therapist.

TEST: The PT can research visible laser light by pointing it to the wall. If the light is uneven and speckled, it is laser light. If there is even light, it is likely to be LED light. Super pulsed lasers cannot be tested this way.
LED light does not have speckles and provides an even impact on tissue.
Recent attention to speckle formation in the tissue has been reported as the phenomenon which sets LLLT apart from other forms of therapeutic light such as light-emitting diodes (LEDs).

This effect, caused by scattered light interference patterns, occurs only with coherent light.

Coherence is a characteristic unique to laser and refers to the light waves being in order or in 'phase' for long trains of up to a meter. This attribute enables a much greater depth of penetration than other forms of light.
The speckle formation also produces local pressure gradients and temperature changes across a cell membrane of .01°C. Although not a perceptible heat change, this causes increased membrane permeability to calcium, sodium and potassium. This can set off a chain reaction of

chemical changes which include increased plasma endorphin and serotonin levels, and reduced bradykinin and C-fibre activity which result in pain relief.

EDITORIAL OVERVIEW

Jan Tunér, closely associated with scientific developments on laser speckles from Hode, has best preferred the description provided by Michael Hamblin from Harvard Medical School for Learners to follow. The speckle phenomenon gives laser therapy an added dimension in treatment potential in new generation research.

PHYSICAL MECHANISMS

According to quantum mechanical theory, light energy is composed of photons or discrete packets of electromagnetic energy. The energy of an individual photon depends only on the wavelength. Therefore, the energy of a "dose" of light depends only on the number of photons and on their wavelength or color (blue photons have more energy than green photons that have more energy than red, that have more energy than NIR, etc). Photons that are delivered into living tissue can either be absorbed or scattered. Scattered photons will eventually be absorbed or will escape from the tissue in the form of diffuse reflection. The photons that are absorbed interact with an organic molecule or chromophore located within the tissue. Because these photons have wavelengths in the red or NIR regions of the spectrum, the chromophores that absorb these photons tend to have delocalized electrons in molecular orbitals that can be excited from the ground state to the first excited state by the quantum of energy delivered by the photon.

According to the first law of thermodynamics, the energy delivered to the tissue must be conserved, and three possible pathways exist to account for what happens to the delivered light energy when low level laser therapy is delivered into tissue.

The commonest pathway that occurs when light is absorbed by living tissue is called internal conversion. This happens when the first excited singlet state of the chromophore undergoes a transition from a higher to a lower electronic state. It is sometimes called "radiationless deexcitation", because no photons are emitted. It differs from intersystem crossing in that, while both are radiationless methods of de-excitation, the molecular spin state for internal conversion remains the same, whereas it changes for intersystem crossing. The energy of the electronically excited state is given off to vibrational modes of the molecule, in other words, the excitation energy is transformed into heat.

The second pathway that can occur is fluorescence. Fluorescence is a luminescence or reemission of light, in which the molecular absorption of a photon triggers the emission of another photon with a longer wavelength. The energy difference between the absorbed and emitted photons ends up as molecular vibrations or heat. The wavelengths involved depend on the absorbance curve and Stokes shift of the particular fluorophore.

The third pathway that can occur after the absorption of light by a tissue chromophore, This represents a number of processes broadly grouped under an umbrella category of photochemistry. Because of the energy of the photons involved, covalent bonds cannot be broken. However, the energy is sufficient for the first excited singlet state to be formed, and this can undergo intersystem crossing to the long-lived triplet state of the chromophore. The long life of this species allows reactions to occur, such as energy transfer to ground state molecular oxygen (a triplet) to form the reactive species, singlet oxygen. Alternatively the chromophore triplet state may undergo electron transfer (probably reduction) to form the radical anion that can then transfer an electron to oxygen to form superoxide. Electron transfer reactions are highly important in the mitochondrial respiratory chain, where the principal chromophores involved in laser therapy are thought to be situated. A third photochemistry pathway that can occur after the absorption of a red or NIR photon is the dissociation of a noncovalently bound ligand from a binding site on a metal containing cofactor in an enzyme. The most likely candidate for this pathway is the binding of nitric oxide to the iron-containing and copper-containing redox canters of the mitochondrial respiratory chain, known as cytochrome c oxidase.

It should be mentioned that there is another mechanism that has been proposed to account for low level laser effects on tissue. This explanation relies on the phenomenon of laser speckle, which is peculiar to laser light. The speckle effect is a result of the interference of many waves, having different phases, which add together to give a resultant wave whose amplitude, and therefore intensity, varies randomly. Each point on illuminated tissue acts as a source of secondary spherical waves. The light at any point in the scattered light field is made up of waves that have been scattered from each point on the illuminated surface. If the surface is rough enough to create path-length differences exceeding one wavelength, giving rise to phase changes greater than 2 , the amplitude (and hence the intensity) of the resultant light varies randomly. It is proposed that the variation in intensity between speckle spots that are about 1 micron apart can give rise to small but steep temperature gradients within subcellular organelles such as mitochondria without causing photochemistry. These temperature gradients are proposed to cause some unspecified changes in mitochondrial metabolism.

Tissue photobiology. The first law of photobiology states that for low power visible light to have any effect on a living biological system, the photons must be absorbed by electronic absorption bands belonging to some molecular chromophore or photo acceptor. One approach to finding the identity of this chromophore is to carry out action spectra. This is a Graph representing biological photo response as a function of wavelength, wave number, frequency, or photon energy, and should resemble the absorption spectrum of the photo acceptor molecule.

The fact that a structured action spectrum can be constructed supports the hypothesis of the existence of cellular photo acceptors and signalling pathways stimulated by light.
The second important consideration involves the optical properties of tissue. Both the absorption and scattering of light in tissue are wavelength dependent (both much higher in the blue region of the spectrum than the red), and the principle tissue chromophore (haemoglobin) has high absorption bands at wavelengths shorter than 600 nm. For these reasons, there is a so called "optical window". The second important consideration involves the optical properties of tissue. Both the absorption and scattering of light in tissue are wavelength dependent (both much higher in the blue region of the spectrum than the red), and the principle tissue chromophores (haemoglobin and melanin) have high absorption bands at wavelengths shorter than 600 nm. Water begins to absorb significantly at wavelengths greater than 1150 nm. For these reasons, there is a so-called "optical window" in tissue covering the red and NIR wavelengths, where the effective tissue penetration of light is maximized. Therefore, although blue, green and yellow light may have significant effects on cells growing in optically transparent culture medium, the use of LLLT in animals and patients almost exclusivelyinvolves red and NIR light (600 - 950 nm).

1.11 PULSING INDICATORS. SP LASERS (GAAs)

Frequencies below recommended are based on empirical evidence are from Jan Tunér, who cautions: Pulsing is effective, due to the deep pulses accumulated over some time. Frequencies are managed additionally but are not the main reasons for the effectiveness of an SP laser treatment.

Pain, neuralgia: 10 – 100 Hz
General stimulation: 700 Hz
Oedema: 1,000 Hz
General stimulation: 2500 Hz
Inflammation: 5000 Hz
Infection: 10,000 Hz
Fig. 1.9

General Rule
When stimulation is required use lower frequencies.
When sedation is required, use higher frequencies.
Treatment frequency and rest time

1.12 NAALT RESEARCH

BIO-EFFECTIVE FEQUENCIES can elicit strong changes in the function of the body, in particular the lower range of frequencies. Frequencies 0.25 – 120 HZ are termed bio effective.

These low frequencies are accepted to be effective in repair and regeneration of tissue, influence immunity response and produce anti-inflammatory effects

BIO SUPPRESSIVE FREQUENCIES can be used to ease pain, reduce inflammation and spasm, and decrease swelling and edema.
These are frequencies of 1000Hz and 3000 Hz

In some cases LLLT may be applied daily if it is convenient and possible. It is most effective due sooner it is used after the injury occurs. On chronic conditions such as arthritis, ringbone, and chips, treatment may be needed for as long as 3 months.

No condition should be continuously treated longer than 3 weeks without a rest period of one week.

Thereafter, treat only every other week, with a one week rest between. As with almost any type of treatment, the body tends to get accustomed to what is happening and begins to ignore the treatment. For this same reason

1.13 CONTINUOUS VS PULSED WAVE MODE

Continuous wave lasers applied on sports related injuries, may generate some heat or warming in tissue. For this reason, PT's prefer SP lasers. Selection of laser is based on the tissue condition and protocol preferred by the therapist.
Use continuous mode for acute conditions.
Generally use 1 - Low setting for chronic conditions.

Change from continuous to pulsing (or vice versa) when:
a) there is no treatment response after a few treatments or
b) Positive progression hits a plateau.

Based on the literature, the following pulsed settings have been used
Option 1 = 1-8 hz for general pain
Option2 = 146 Hz General Stimulation, Trigger points
Option3 = 1000 Hz Edema, Inflammation

You can only offer pulsing frequencies that your Lasers is programmed to. Research has indicated that the progression of light absorption in tissue is linear with SP lasers, whilst continuous with CW lasers. SP lasers deliver strong pulses of laser light into the skin faster than CW lasers. Skin penetration of profiles of different lasers, on different skin photo types, and with different treatment modes are a subject of scientific enquiry.

Editorial selections from a prominent WALT group

In clinical practice, the different skin penetration profiles for super pulsed and continuous lasers will have some clinical implications. In addition to different optimal doses as reflected in WALT guidelines, the penetration profile influences skin temperature during LLLT treatment.

We found lower thermal effects in dark skin from 904nm super pulsed laser than from 810nm continuous laser in one of our earlier studies. This difference in thermal effects from these two lasers can be explained by skin penetration profile. The percentage of energy absorbed in skin during processing time is decreased for super pulsed lasers, whereas it is constant for continuous lasers. In addition, 904nm super pulsed lasers have better skin penetration initially than do 810nmcontinuous lasers.

Tuner: The pigment in hair absorbs the laser energy locally and for persons with dark hair, the laser can even produce a burning sensation, so I move the probe in a circle in these areas to avoid pain.

Laser therapy effects can be influenced by body temperature. This means LOCAL body temperature, for instance in an inflamed area where there is edema and consequently more blood, absorbing the energy. So it is not a straightforward answer to the question whether body temperature influences laser therapy. A body temp of 37 or 38 degrees makes no difference.

1.13 COMPREHENSIVE TREATMENT

A comprehensive treatment approach results in more rapid, successful outcomes (Generally a minimum of 2 approaches should be used). Assessment, diagnosis and testing results will determine which of the following areas require treatment:

Nerve root or superficial nerve trunks
Entire injured or affected area
Motor or trigger points
Referred areas of pain
Acupuncture and / or auricular points

For extensive oedema, treat proximal (centrally) to distal (towards extremities),to open up the lymphatic pathway to enhance drainage. Drain the master node before and after the session.

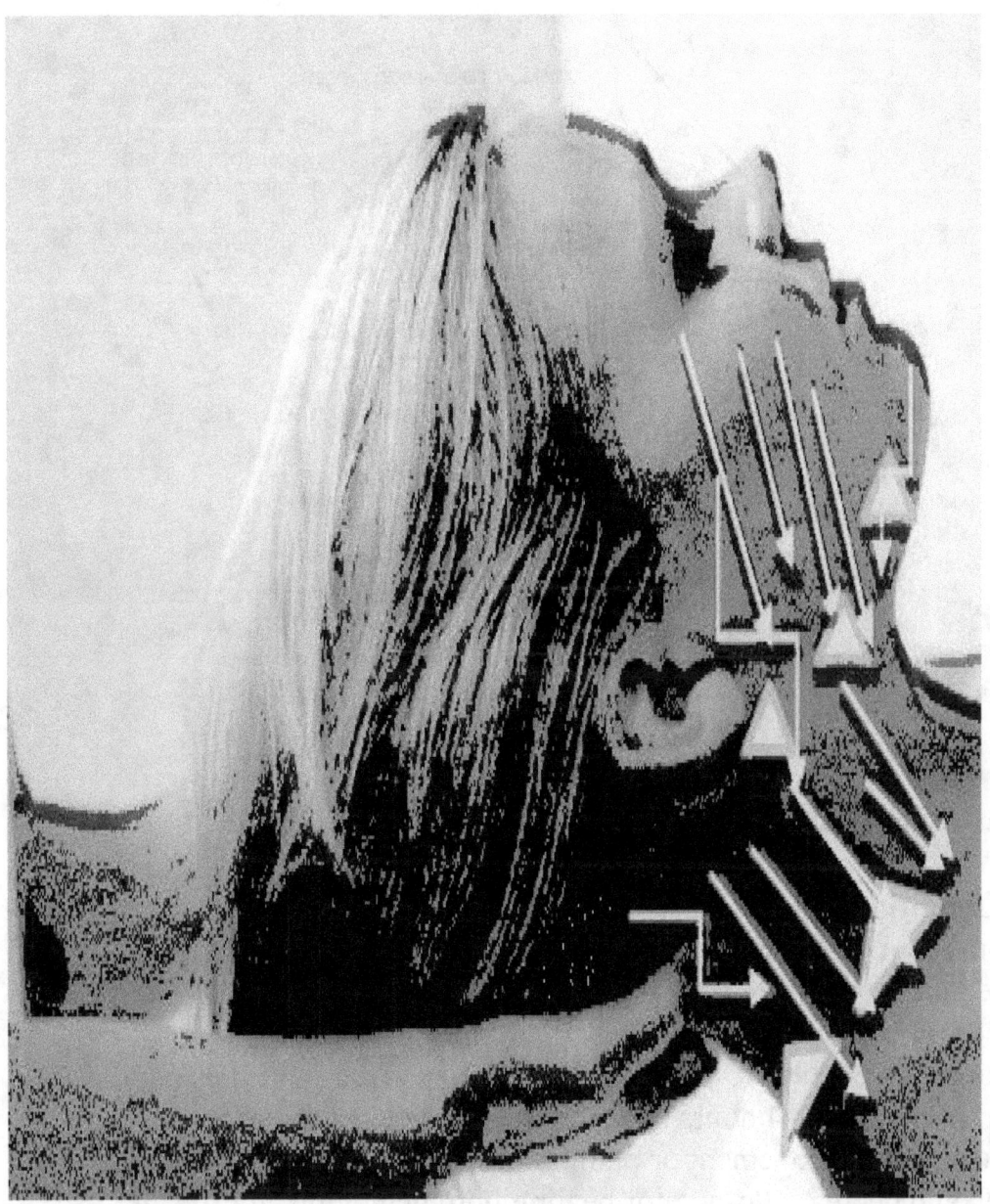

1.14 TREATMENT STEPS

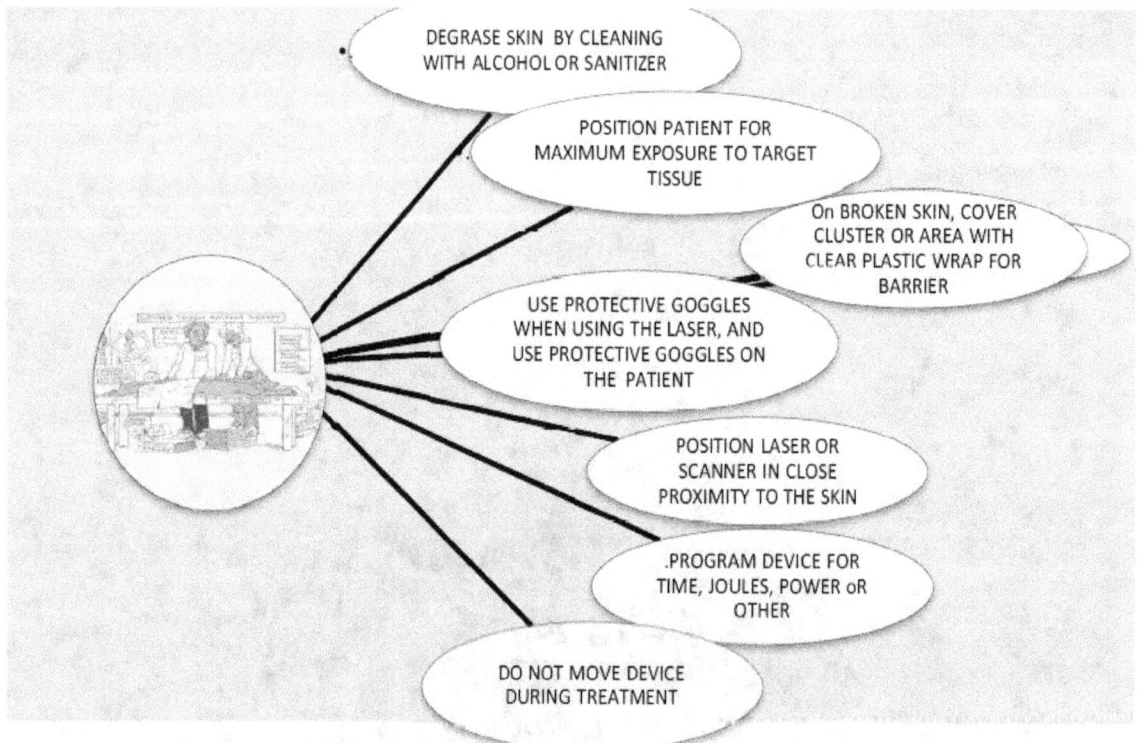

1.15 TREATMENT GUIDELINES

Treatment Schedule

Acute Conditions - Treat daily to 3 times weekly until significant
Symptom relief is achieved, especially for patients with trauma,
Herniated discs and acute back pain. Treatment may last
1-3 weeks with 6-15 treatments.
With competitive athletes, treatment may be delivered 2-3 times per day
With a minimum of 2-4 hours between sessions, for rapid response.
Once sufficient improvement or pain relief is achieved, treat 2-3 times
Per week and decrease dosage for healing until achieving significant
Improvement or full resolution.

Chronic Conditions - Treat 2-3 times weekly Up to 15-25 treatments.
Maintenance treatment may be required for chronic degenerative conditions.

Consistent schedule of treatments augment the accumulative effects enhancing outcomes.

Occasionally, pain can increase following the first few treatments,

DEGRASE SKIN BY CLEANING
   •. WITH ALCOHOL OR SANITIZER
POSITION PATIENT FOR
MAXIMUM EXPOSURE TO TARGET TISSUE
   •. On BROKEN SKIN, COVER
CLUSTER OR AREA WITH
CLEAR PLASTIC WRAP FOR BARRIER
   • USE PROTECTIVE GOGGLES
WHEN USING THE LASER, AND
USE PROTECTIVE GOGGLES ON THE PATIENT
   • POSITION LASER OR
SCANNER IN CLOSE PROXIMITY TO THE SKIN.
PROGRAM DEVICE FOR TIME, JOULES, POWER OR OTHER
   • DO NOT MOVE DEVICE DURING TREATMENT

(2 - 4 hours post treatment until the next day).

This is referred to as a 'treatment reaction', an indication that the light energy may have "pushed" the chronic condition into a sub-acute phase of healing. Forewarn patients so ice or analgesics can be used. Once this pain subsides, pain levels are generally less than pre-treatment ratings.

Next session, decrease treatment dose by 50%and gradually increase over time.

Frail individuals, small children and patients with degenerative rheumatoid arthritis, fibromyalgia or other autoimmune conditions should be treated initially with smaller doses.

Gradually work up to full dosage.

Patients are frequently assessed and discharged when response is adequate.

1.16 USE OF OTHER MODALITIES

Other Physiotherapy modalities may be unnecessary with phototherapy.

If combining modalities, treatment sequence is important:

If icing, use before phototherapy

(Vasoconstriction decreases blood flow, improving light penetration).

If massage or heat generating therapy (e.g. ultrasound, e-stim) is used, apply after phototherapy.
(Vasodilation increases blood flow, diminishing penetration of light).

1.17 WALT GUIDELINES (no claims made)

Physical therapy may be approached with super pulsed or continuous wave lasers where the mean output of power is less than 500mw or FDA cleared 3b or lower. A chopped, pulsed laser is not preferred for therapy, but considered a modification of a CW laser.
Guidelines for doses are recommended by World Association for Laser Therapy (WALT) which have been compiled during meta-analysis. Emphasis is that the Physical Therapist follows the overall power output of the laser.

Dose recommendations are starting points and not cook book formulas. Doses may be lowered or increased depending upon patient's response.
The Physical Therapist must follow the Arndt Schultz Principle indicating that weak stimuli activate physiological processes, and very strong stimuli inhibit physiological responses.

For SP Lasers, normal doses range between 1 J/sq cm and 4J/sq cm.
For CW lasers the range is between 4J/sq cm and16 J/sq cm. The difference in doses is attributed to the greater power density of Super Pulsed lasers which thus allows smaller doses. This provides a dosimetry range from lower to higher.

WALT guidelines – (discussed further in Section 3)

SUPER PULSED LASERS
Stimulatory dose for repair. Low. 1 – 2 J/sq. cm
Medium 2 – 3 J/sq. cm
Inhibitory dose for pain High 3 – 4 J/sq. cm
CONTINUOUS WAVELASER 785, 808, 830 nm
Stimulatory dose for repair. Low 6 – 8 J/sq. cm
Medium 8 -12 J/sq. cm. Inhibitory dose for pain. High 12 – 16 J/ sq.

FUTURISTIC LIGHT

LLLT has enormous potential in energy medicine based on ongoing discoveries, providing scope for drugless healing

-Modification of light effects with chemicals. Karu

****Research has shown that chemicals may be used to lower the receptivity of light or to increase the receptivity of light. Chlorophyll is a photosensitizer that increases the action spectra of laser light. Reducing agents of the respiratory chain, sodium dithionite, inhibits the reception of laser light.

Chemical usage is significant in photodynamic therapy in the treatment of tumours

- The infinite possibilities of the mitochondria with irradiation. Karu

-**** The mitochondria might play a role in regulating the expression of several genes in the nucleus. This involves the existence of a signalling pathway from the mitochondrion to the nucleus. The mitochondrion contains 5-10 identical, circular molecules of DNA, each of which carries information for 37 genes. Gene discovery studies documented a significant up regulation of gene expression pathways involved in mitochondrial energy production and antioxidant cellular protection. These findings

indicated links to the action of red to near IR radiation on mitochondrial oxidative metabolism and changes in cell response to the irradiation.

Mitochondria have not only life supporting (even developments of a mitochondria ultrastructure under specific irradiation schemes), but also death promoting functions. This factor has to be considered when stimulating cell metabolism via activation of the respiratory Chain.

Mitochondrial structural transformations, and giant mitochondria are potentials for high levels of respiration and energy turnover that can transfer energy along extensive mitochondrial membranes, which further connect remote cell regions to level out the gradients of energy

yielding and energy consuming components. This hypothesis makes possible the assumption that the formation of the giant mitochondria in lymphocytes subject to irradiation provides energy for the process needed for nucleus reactivation.

THIS LITERATURE IS BASED ON EMPIRICAL EVIDENCE FROM META ANALAYSIS
OF PUBLISHED RESEARCH, SUBMISSIONS FROM WALT, NAALT, TUNÉR HODE,

PROF .PONTINEN, OSHIRO, KARU- IMPORTANT LASER THERAPY
BOOKS AND
COURSES, AND CONGRESS PAPERS
**All editorial insights and contributions belong to Jan Tunér on recent
literature status of LLLT**

SECTION TWO

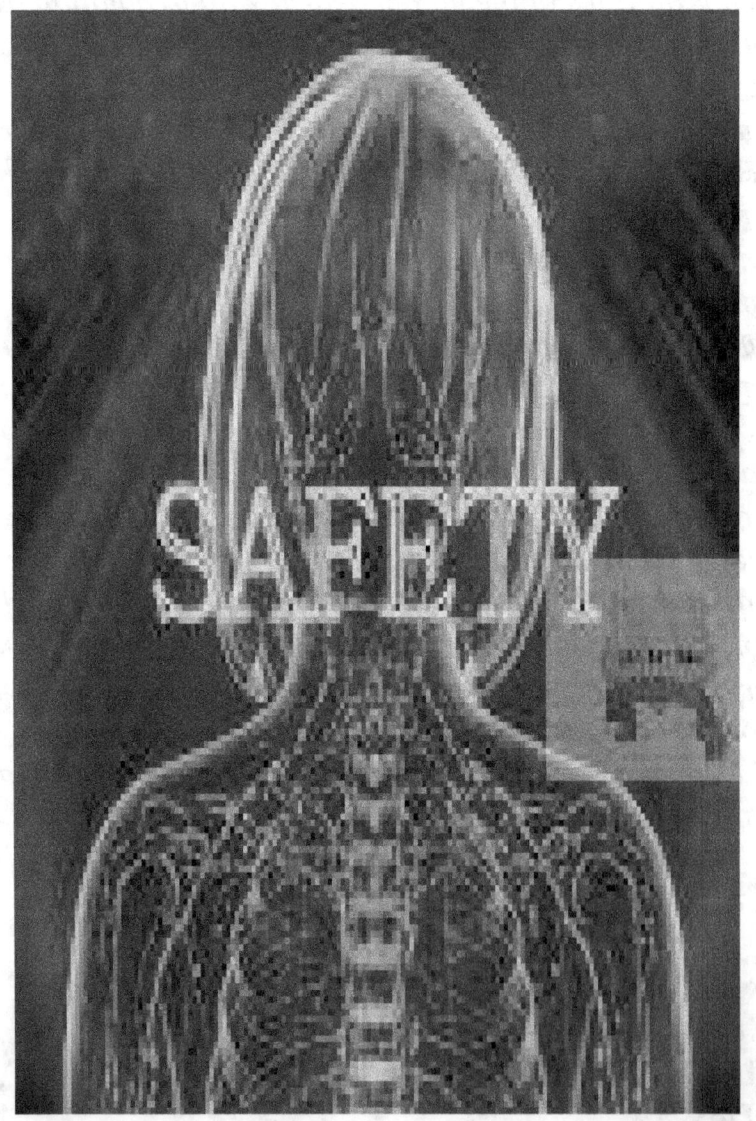

OSHA, ANSI AND FDA STANDARDSAND OCCUPATIONAL SAFETY

SECTION TWO

SKILLS DEVELOPMENT IN THIS SECTION

UNDERSTANDING OF LASER SAFETY
PRACTICAL MANAGEMENT OF LASER SAFETY
FDA RECOMMENDATIONS
SAFETY IN OWN PRACTISE

CONTENTS

2.1 LASER CLASSES

Lasers and laser systems are assigned one of four broad Classes (I to IV) depending on the potential for causing biological damage. The biological basis of the hazard classes are summarized below.

Class I: cannot emit laser radiation at known hazard levels (typically continuous wave: CW 0.4µW at visible wavelengths). Users of Class I laser products are generally exempt from radiation hazard controls during operation and maintenance (but not necessarily during service).
Since lasers are not classified on beam access during service, most Class I industrial lasers will consist of a higher class (high power) controls are recommended. Laser enclosed in a properly interlocked and labelled protective enclosure. In some cases, the enclosure may be a room
(walk-in protective housing) which requires a means to prevent operation when operators are inside the room.

Class I.A: a special designation that is based upon a 1000-second exposure and applies only to lasers that are "not intended for viewing" such as a supermarket laser scanner. The upper power limit of Class I.A. is 4.0 mw. The emission from a Class I.A. laser is defined such that the emission does not exceed the Class I limit for an emission duration of 1000 seconds.

Class II: low-power visible lasers that emit above Class I levels but at a radiant power not above 1 mw. The concept is that the human aversion reaction to bright light will protect a person.
Only limited controls are specified.

Class IIIA: intermediate power lasers (CW: 1-5 mw). Only hazardous for intrabeam viewing.
Some limited controls are usually recommended.

NOTE: There are different logotype labelling requirements for Class IIIA lasers with a beam irradiance that does not exceed 2.5 mw/cm2 (Caution logotype) and those where the beam irradiance does exceed 2.5 mw/cm2 (Danger logotype).

Class IIIB: moderate power lasers (CW: 5-500 mw/1000mw, pulsed: 10 J/cm2 or the diffuse reflection limit, whichever is lower). In general Class IIIB lasers will not be a fire hazard, nor are they generally capable of producing a hazardous diffuse reflection.

Class IV: High power lasers (CW: 500 mw, pulsed: 10 J/cm2 or the diffuse reflection limit) are hazardous to view under any condition (directly or diffusely scattered).

These lasers have Area potential fire hazard and a skin hazard. Significant controls are required of Class IV laser facilities.

2.2. LASER CLASSIFICATIONS--SUMMARY OF HAZARDS

Class	Applies to wavelength ranges				Hazards		
	UV	VIS	NIR	IR	Direct ocular	Diffuse ocular	Fire
I	X	X	X	X	No	No	No
IA	--	X*	--	--	Only after 1000 sec	No	No
II	--	X	--	--	Only after 0.25 sec	No	No
IIIA	X	X**	X	X	Yes	No	No
IIIB	X	X	X	X	Yes	Only when laser output is near Class IIIB limit of 0.5 Watt	No
IV	X	X	X	X	Yes	Yes	Yes

Key:
X = Indicates class applies in wavelength range.
* = Class IA applicable to lasers "not intended for viewing" ONLY.
** = CDRH Standard assigns Class IIIA to visible wavelengths ONLY. ANSI Z 136.1 assigns Class IIIA to all wavelength ranges.

It should be stressed that classification is a required specification provided by the laser manufacturer and the label that specifies the class is found in only one location on the laser product. The class of the laser will be specified only on the lower left-hand corner (position three) of the warning logotype label.

The logotype is the rectangular label that has the laser "sunburst" symbol and the warning statement of CAUTION (Class II and some Class IIIA) or DANGER (some Class IIIA, all Class IIIB and Class IV). This label will also have the type of laser designated (HeNe, Argon, CO2, etc.) and the power or energy output specified (1 mw CW/MAX, 100 mj pulsed, etc.). Class I lasers have no required labelling indicating the Class I status.

2.3 OPTICAL FIBER SERVICE GROUP DESIGNATIONS.

Optical Fibre Communication Systems (OFCS) and the associated optical test sets use semiconductor lasers or LED transmitters that emit energy at wavelengths typically in the range from 0.650 to 1.20 mm into the light-guide fibre-optic cables.

Under the requirements of the FLPPS, the manufacturer is first required to classify the laser as either a Class-I, Class-II, Class-I.A., Class-IIIA, Class-IIIB, or Class-IV laser product and then to certify (by means of a label on the product) as well as submit a report demonstrating that all requirements (performance features) of the compliance standard are met.

Specific performance features include:

1. protective housing;
2. protective housing warning and logotype labels;
3. product identification label and certification statement;
4. safety interlocks;
5. emission indicator;
6. remote interlock connector;
7. key control;

8. beam attenuator;
9. specification of control locations;
10. viewing optic limitations;
11. scanning beam safeguards; and
12. manual reset of beam cut off.

The American National Standard Institute (ANSI). An American National Standard implies a consensus of those substantially concerned with its scope and provisions. These standards are intended as a guide for manufacturers, consumers. Compliance is voluntary unless specifically required by an organization.

FOR THE PRACTITIONER

Since laser apparatus comes from many countries and manufacturers, it is important to check on the positioning of the logo, the safety sign, the security of the outer cover and operating instructions or controls. Safety is the most important criterion for clinical use.

2.4 PERMISSABLE LASER EXPOSURE LIMITS

At present either the FDA criteria for medical lasers or the following ANSI standards can be useful in evaluating laser safety.

Maximum Permissible Exposure Limits.

A summary of Maximum Permissible Exposure (MPE) limits for direct ocular exposures for some of the more common lasers is presented below. The information below provides the MPE value for different lasers operating for different overall exposure times. The times chosen were

0.25 second: The human aversion time for bright-light stimuli (the blink reflex). Thus, this becomes the "first line of defence" for unexpected exposure to some lasers and is the basis of the Class II concept.

10 seconds: The time period chosen by the ANSI Z 136.1 committees represents the optimum "worst-case" time period for ocular exposures to

infrared (principally near-infrared) laser sources. It was argued that natural eye motions dominate for periods longer than 10 seconds.

600 seconds: The time period chosen by the ANSI Z 136.1 committees represents a typical worst-case period for viewing visible diffuse reflections during tasks such as alignment.

30,000 seconds: The time period that represents a full 1-day (8-hour) occupational exposure. This results from computing the number of seconds in 8 hours; e.g.: 8 hours × 60 minutes/hour × 60 seconds/minute = 28,800 seconds. Rounded off, it becomes 30,000 seconds.

b. The "safety" exposure limits (MPE's) are expressed in irradiance terms (W/cm2) that would be measured at the cornea. Note that they vary by wavelength and exposure time.

2.5 FDA/CDRH REQUIREMENTS FOR LASER PRODUCTS

```
----------- Class1 -----------
Requirements              I   IA   II   IIIB   IV
Performance (all laser products)
Protective housing        R2  R2   R2   R2  R2   R2
Safety interlock          R3,4 R3,4 R3,4 R3,4 R3,4 R3,4
Location of controls _    R   R  _  R      R
Viewing optics            R   R    R    R    R    R
Scanning safeguard        R   R    R    R    R    R
Performance (laser systems)
Remote control connector _ _ _           _ R      R
Key control _ _ _ _                        R      R
Emission indicator _      _       R    R    R10    R10
Beam attenuator _                 R    R    R      R
Reset _ _ _ _ _                                    R13

Performance (specific purpose products)
```

Medical	S	S	S	S8	S8	S8
Surveying, levelling, alignment	S	S	S	S	NP	NP
Demonstration	S	S	S	S	S11	S11
Labelling (all laser products)						
Certification and identification	R	R	R	R	R	R
Aperture _ _			R	R	R	R
Class warning	R6	R7	R9	R12	R12	
User information	R	R	R	R	R	R
Product literature _		R	R	R	R	R
Service information	R	R	R	R	R	R

Key: R= required

_   not applicable

S̄   =same as other products of class

NP   =not permitted

D   =depends on level of interior radiation.

Notes:
1. Based on highest level accessible during operation.
2. Required wherever and whenever human access to laser radiation above Class I limits is not needed for product to perform its function.
3. Required for protective housings opened during operation or maintenance, if human access thus gained is not
4. always necessary when housing is opened. Interlock requirements vary according to Class of internal radiation.
5. Wording depends on level and wavelength of laser radiation within protective housing.
6. Warning statement label.
7. CAUTION logotype.
8. Requires means to measure level of radiation intended to irradiate the body.
9. CAUTION if 2.5 mWcm-2 or less, DANGER if greater than 2.5 mWcm-2.
10. Delay required between indication and emission.
11. Variance required for Class IIIB or IV demonstration laser products and
12. Light shows.
13. DANGER logotype.
14. Required after August 20, 1986.

THE AMERICAN NATIONAL STANDARDS INSTITUTE (ANSI).

An American National Standard implies a consensus of those substantially concerned with its scope and provisions. These standards are intended as a guide to aid the manufacturer, the consumer and the general public. There is, however, no inherent requirement for anyone or any company to adhere to an ANSI standard. At present, the following ANSI standards can be useful.

2.6 SOME DISPLAY SIGNS FOR OCCUPATIONAL SAFETY
WARNING SIGNS

Below are some signs used on lasers and clinics where laser therapy sessions take place –
CAUTION

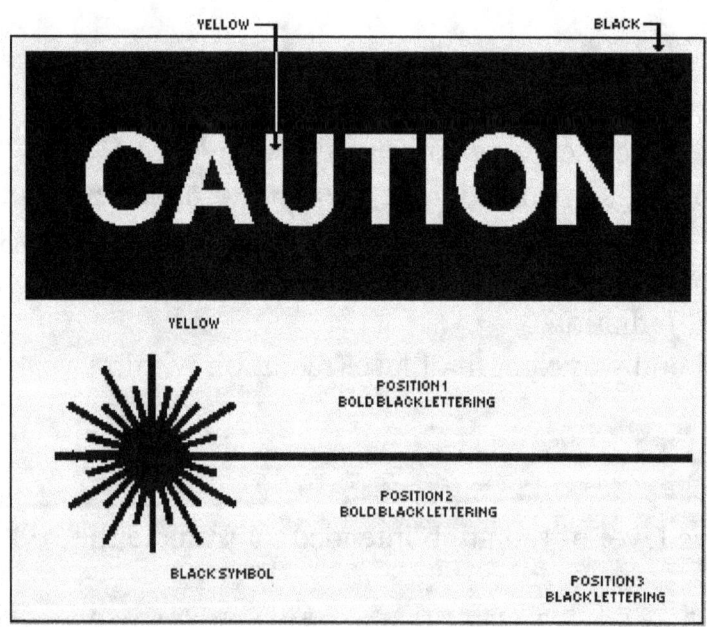

DANGER

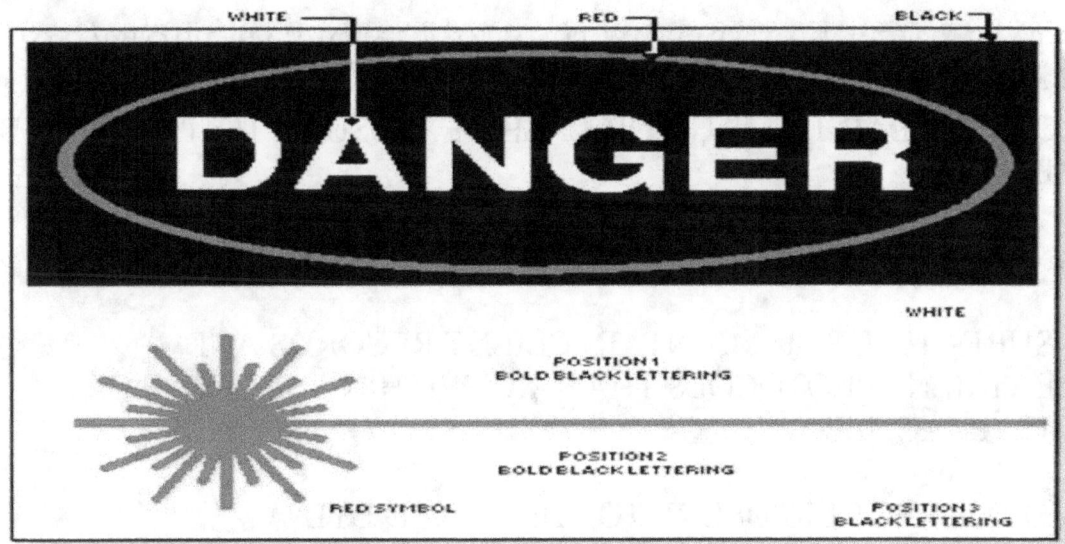

LASER REPAIR NOTICE

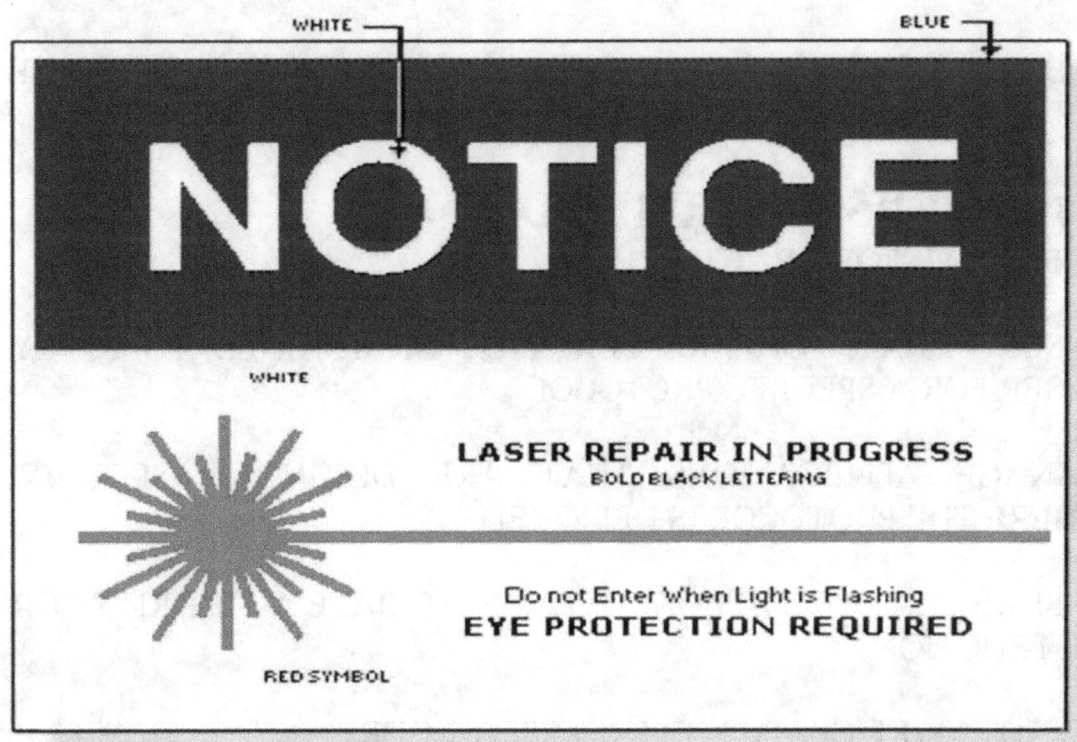

2.7 MORE ON SAFETY

OBTAIN THE CLIENTS WRITTEN CONSENTWEAR PROTECTIVE GLASSES CERTIFIED TO PROTECT CLIENT AND THERAPIST FROM OCULAR DAMAGE OR LASER EXPOSURE TO THE NAKED EYE

SANITIZE YOUR LASER BEFORE AND AFTER TREATMENTS

ENSURE THAT YOU MAINTAIN CLIENT RECORDS AND TREATMENT PROTOCOLS THAT ARE WITHIN THE SCOPE OF YOUR PRACTISE

AVOID DIRECT EXPOSURE TO THE NAKED EYE

AVOID DIRECT RADIATION ON A FETUS, OR ON THE FETUS AREA OF A PREGNANT WOMAN

AVOID EXPOSING PATIENTS WHO ARE HYPERSENSITIVE TO LIGHT

UPDATE YOUR LASER SKILLS THROUGH GENUINE INSTRUCTORS

2.8 LASERS AND THE FDA
APPROVAL FOR PRACTISE

ENSURE THAT YOU ARE CERTIFIED OR TRAINED TO APPLY LASER FOR A SPECIFIC PROTOCOL

MANAGE APPLICATIONS THAT ARE DIAGNOSIS SPECIFIC: WHERE THE PROTOCOL IS DESIGNED

ENSURE THAT YOU BELONG TO A LEGITIMATE AUTHORITY FOR INSTRUCTION

DO NOT MAKE CLAIMS OR PROMISE TO CURE

DOCUMENT ALL PROCEDURES AND RECORDS

MANAGE ORGANIZATIONAL SKILLS

MANAGE COMMUNICATION SKILLS TO INFORM THE CLIENT

STAY UPDATED IN RESEARCH AND SCIENTIFIC LITERATURE

2.9 NATIONAL OCCUPATIONAL STANDARDS

These are global standards in organizational safety which give security to individuals and groups locating or receiving therapy when they live or travel away from their native homelands.

SAFETY IN PHYSICAL THERAPY

- Manage your own practice to be with minimal risk.

- Assess risk in your workplace and take timely remedial measures.

- Do not delay treatments. Practise Time Management and effective treatment strategies that engender client trust and confidence.

- Obtain documented feedback of client satisfaction and ensure steps are taken to assess reasons for dissatisfaction in clients.

- Do not use a laser that is not functioning due to broken lens, low battery, Faulty electric wiring or other.

- Document standard operating procedures for Safety Assessment of laser

- Safety assessment of workplace including environmental, ventilation, room temperatures, hygiene and sanitization factors or other.

- Client assessment and records, including arrangements for client referral to other medical departments if needed

- Workplace arrangements for CARE if required

- Treatment protocols of any laser treatment that are within the scope of your practice

- Assess your own practice, and take measures to remain up to date as attending seminars, reading news books and researching the internet.

- If affordable, update your own laser.

- Maintain 'Equality in Diversity' in your practice. Do not exhibit racial, socio economic, caste, creed or other barriers in your practice. This permits 'social security' in your clinic.

- Manage your clinic with effective organizational safety systems as fire control, theft control, safety of data and records, security within the premises. Ensure that your organization employees are trained in reporting and managing hazards.

Occupational Standards of Competence in Physical Therapy are developed In two aspects. These are

1) Professional Practice

2) Patient/Client Management

These are discussed below.

2.10 STANDARDS OF COMPETENCE IN PROFESSIONAL PRACTISE(in Laser therapy)

1) PROFESSIONAL ACCOUNTABILITY
The physical therapist:

• Practices in a safe manner that minimizes risk to patients, self and others.

• Completes documentation related to physical therapy practice in an appropriate, legible, and timely manner that is consistent with all applicable laws and regulatory requirements.

• Supervises assistive personnel and students in a manner that assures safe and efficient care.

• Consistently and critically evaluates sources of information related to physical therapy practice, outcomes research and education and applies knowledge from these sources in a scientific manner and to appropriate populations.

• Selects and utilizes outcomes measures to assess the results of interventions administered to individual and groups of patients.

• Communicates effectively with clients, caregivers and professional colleagues.

2) PROFESSIONAL BEHAVIOR

The physical therapist:

• Conducts critical self-assessment in order to practice to the fullest extent of knowledge, skills and abilities and takes responsibility to make accommodations as necessary.

• Demonstrates an understanding of and compliance with all laws and regulations governing the practice of physical therapy in his/her jurisdiction.

• Forms a professional relationship with patients/clients, colleagues and other members of the health care team in an effort to maximize patient/client outcomes.

• Avoids potential conflict of interest situations and circumstances that could be construed as harassment or abuse of patients, colleagues, associates or employees.

• Demonstrates sensitivity to individual and cultural differences when engaged in physical therapy practice

• Demonstrates knowledge and works to accommodate health disparities for individuals and the community at large.

LOW LEVEL LASER THERAPY FOR PHYSICAL THERAPISTS

3) PROFESSIONAL DEVELOPMENT

The physical therapist:

• Demonstrates lifelong learning to identify, acquire and apply knowledge, skills and abilities required for current physical therapy practice.

• Develops the knowledge, skills and abilities to communicate, manage knowledge, mitigate error and support decision-making utilizing information technology

STANDARDS OF COMPETENCE IN PATIENT/CLIENT MANAGEMENT (In relevance to laser therapy)

1) EXAMINATION, EVALUATION AND DIAGNOSIS

The physical therapist:

• Consistently integrates the best evidence for practice from all sources of information and utilizes clinical judgment to determine the best care for a patient.

• Safely examines a patient/client using valid and reliable measures whenever available.

• Establishes a diagnosis and prognosis for physical therapy, identifies risks of care, and makes appropriate clinical decisions based upon the examination and evaluation, including history, screening and differential diagnosis, and current available evidence.

• Identifies and considers patient/client goals and expected outcomes.

• Discusses findings with and obtains consent from the patient/client prior to commencing any physical therapy intervention.

• When appropriate, refers the patient/client to colleagues or other members of the health care team.

2) PLAN OF CARE

The physical therapist:

• Establishes and monitors a plan of care in consultation, cooperation and collaboration with the patient/client and other involved health care team members to insure that care is continuous and reliable.

• Evaluates and updates the plan of care as indicated based on the patient\client status, results of psychometrically valid outcomes measures when available, and applicable laws and regulations.

• Incorporates appropriate, timely and efficient use of resources (environmental, equipment, care-giver support and financial) when establishing a plan of care.

3) IMPLEMENTATION
The physical therapist:
• Delivers, evaluates and adjusts the physical therapy intervention.
• Takes appropriate action in any emergency situation.
• Utilizes assistive personnel in accordance with legal requirements.

4) EDUCATION

The physical therapist:

• Educates patients/clients, family, and caregivers, using relevant and effective teaching methods to assure optimal patient care outcomes.

5) DISCHARGE

The physical therapist:

• Plans for discharge in consultation with the patient/client and care givers.

• Discharges the patient/client after expected outcomes have been achieved or documents rationale for discharge when outcomes have not been achieved.

• Assists in the coordination of ongoing care if required.

ORGANIZATIONAL SAFETY

Manage the Housekeeping - the assembling, sorting, simplifying, highlighting, sustaining and securing structures in the organization of all process, document, personnel and network.

Safety of data maintenance, is as important as the safety from assessing risk through a certified assessor and finding arrangements to reduce the risk.

Organizational policy must secure personnel and financial strength in means, back up and support through efficient training and network.

9. COMMANDMENTS ABOUT SAFETY

Everybody is responsible for own and others safety in the workplace

All accidents are preventable

Follow company policies

Assess the risks. Stop and think.

Be proactive in Safety

Don't take shortcuts

Get trained support

Be prepared

Review daily. Manage internal and external audits especially at times of change.

HIGHLIGHTS

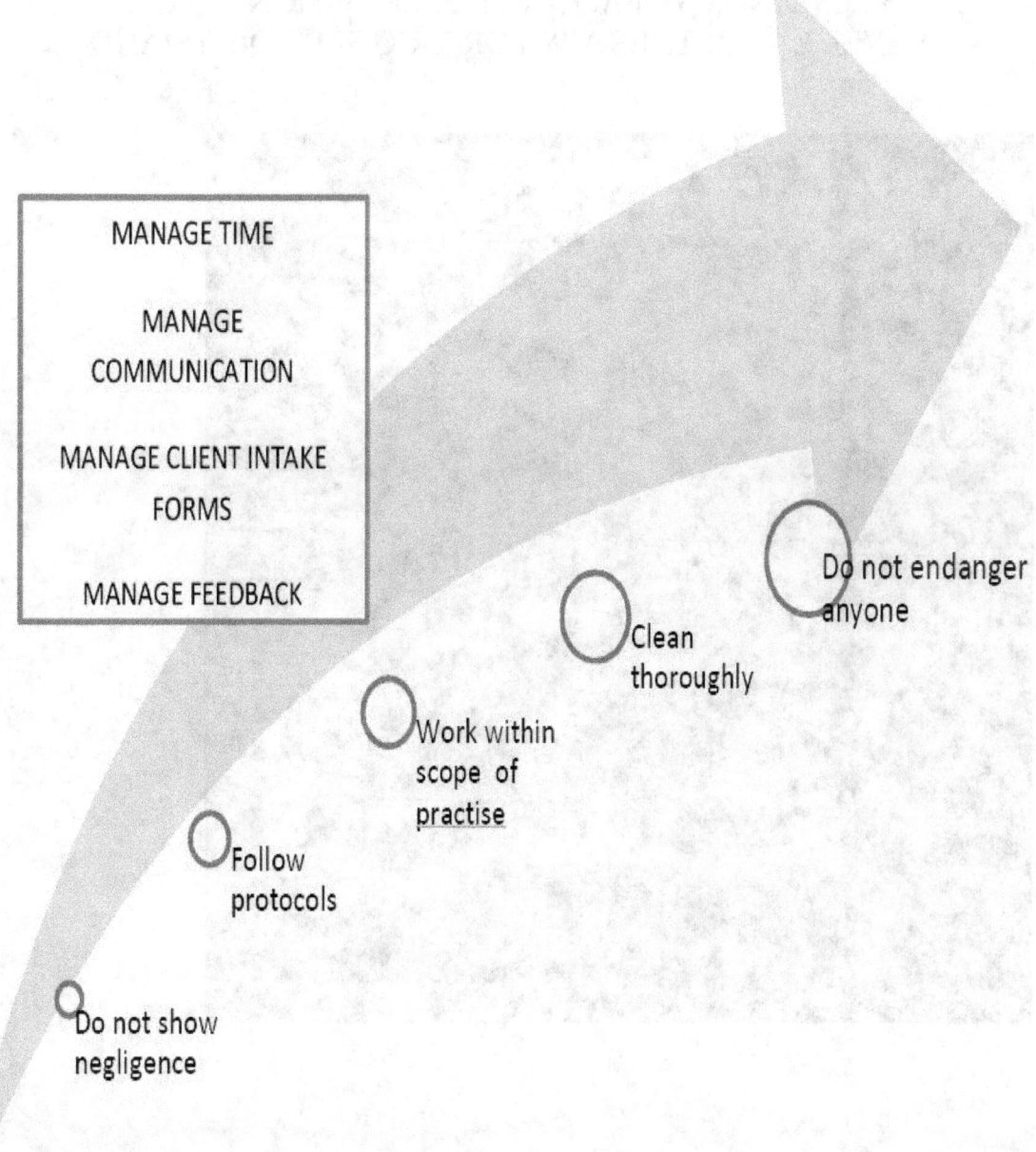

MANAGE TIME

MANAGE COMMUNICATION

MANAGE CLIENT INTAKE FORMS

MANAGE FEEDBACK

Do not endanger anyone

Clean thoroughly

Work within scope of practise

Follow protocols

Do not show negligence

SECTION 3

MYOFASCIAL RELEASE WITH LOW LEVEL LASER THERAPY
>UNDERSTANDING THE ANATOMY OF THE MYOFASCIAL SYSTEM
>UNDERSTANDINGMYOFASCIAL DYSFUNCTION
>LOW LEVEL LASER THERAPY FOR TRIGGER POINTS AND

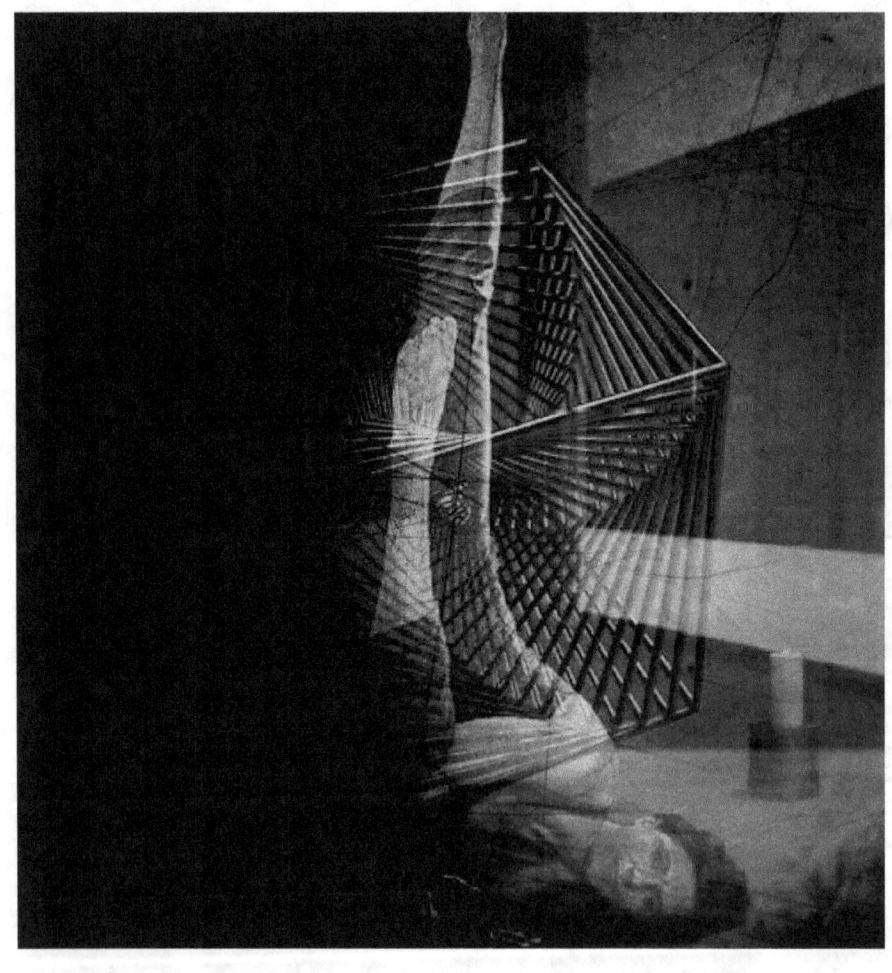

MYOFASCIAL RELEASE

SKILLS DEVELOPMENT IN THIS SECTION

KNOWING THE FASCIA AND ITS DYSFUNCTIONAL PATTERN
APPLYING TRIGGER POINT THERAPY USING LLLT
DEVELOPING TREATMENT PROTOCOLS FOR PT
FOLLOWING WALT GUIDELINES

CONTENT

3.1 MYOFASCIAL ANATOMY

Fascia, is a connective tissue that is continuous throughout the body, and is considered the 'skeleton' of soft tissue. It is pervasive, encompassing nerves, muscles, lymph vessels, organs, the brain and more.

Fascia serves the following functions
1) It forms and supports. It gives shape to the body and its component parts and holds them in place
2) It restricts. By providing firm boundaries it improves muscle strength. Muscles without fascia are considerably weaker.
3) It guides and moulds. Damaged bone deprived of periosteum (fascia) does not heal appropriately. In bad cases it can form adhesions between structures and alter healthy tissue.
4) It contains and compartmentalizes. Fascia contains and channels body fluids, helping to prevent infection from spreading.
5) It provides infrastructure for branching systems. It supports capillaries and vessels of the circulatory and lymphatic systems, as well as the ubiquitous branching of the nervous system.
6) It gives rise to new connective tissue. It contains fibroblasts, proliferated by low level laser to thicken connective tissue, repair tendons, ligaments, stimulate growth factor and re densify impaired tissue.

3.2 SUPERFICIAL OR DEEP FASCIA

SUPERFICIAL FASCIA

The superficial fascia is also called the hypodermis, sub cutis, or stratum subcutaneum. It is located directly under the skin and contains fat, fascicles of muscle tissue, cutaneous blood vessels and nerves, and about half of the fat in the body.
Superficial laser beams and LEDS penetrate this tissue.

DEEP FASCIA

The deep fascia is all of the fascia that is deep to the superficial fascia, with which it is continuous. Deep fascia includes the fascia covering a group of muscles, the epimysium which surrounds the muscles, and the perimysium which surrounds the fascicles within the muscle, and the endomysium which surround the individual muscle fibres. Each layer gives rise to the next deep layer, imposing limits on muscle contractile force and giving indications of muscle tension.

CW and Super pulsed IR lasers penetrate this tissue.

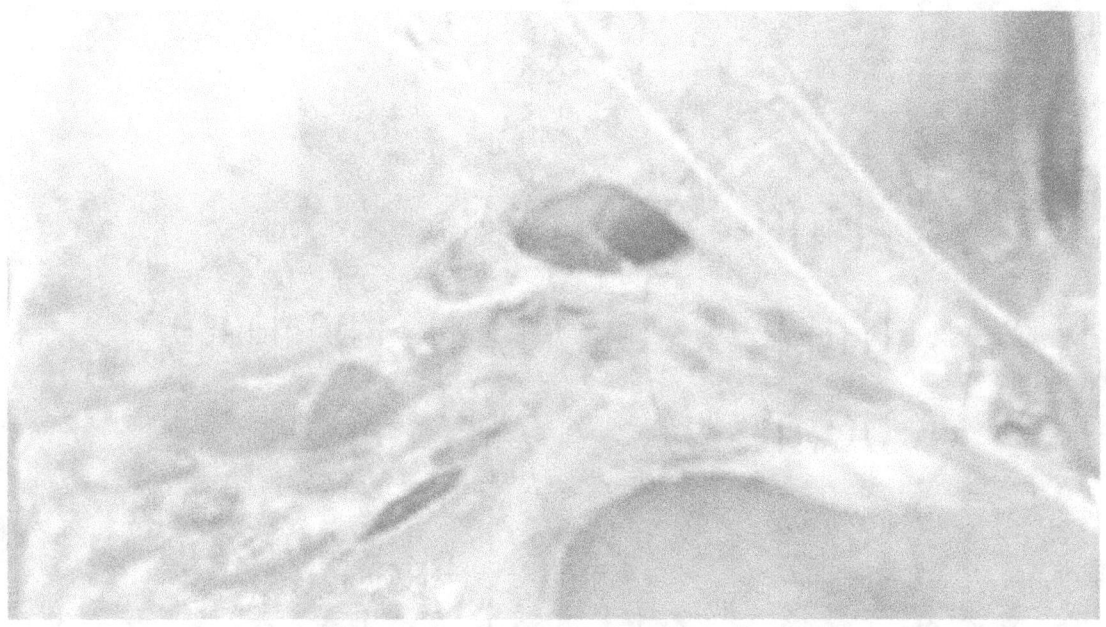

From Luigi Stecco, Carla Stecco - 'Fascial manipulation. Practical part'

3.3 MYOFASCIAL DYSFUNCTION

Physical therapists must know how to assess fascia as an indication of health or sickness, through deep knowledge and understanding of human anatomy. Patients whose fascia behaves abnormally in acute or chronic conditions are considered to be with myo fascial dysfunction.

Low level laser is an effective tool to correct myo fascial dysfunction in a very short time.

INDICATIONS OF MYOFASCIAL DYSFUNCTION

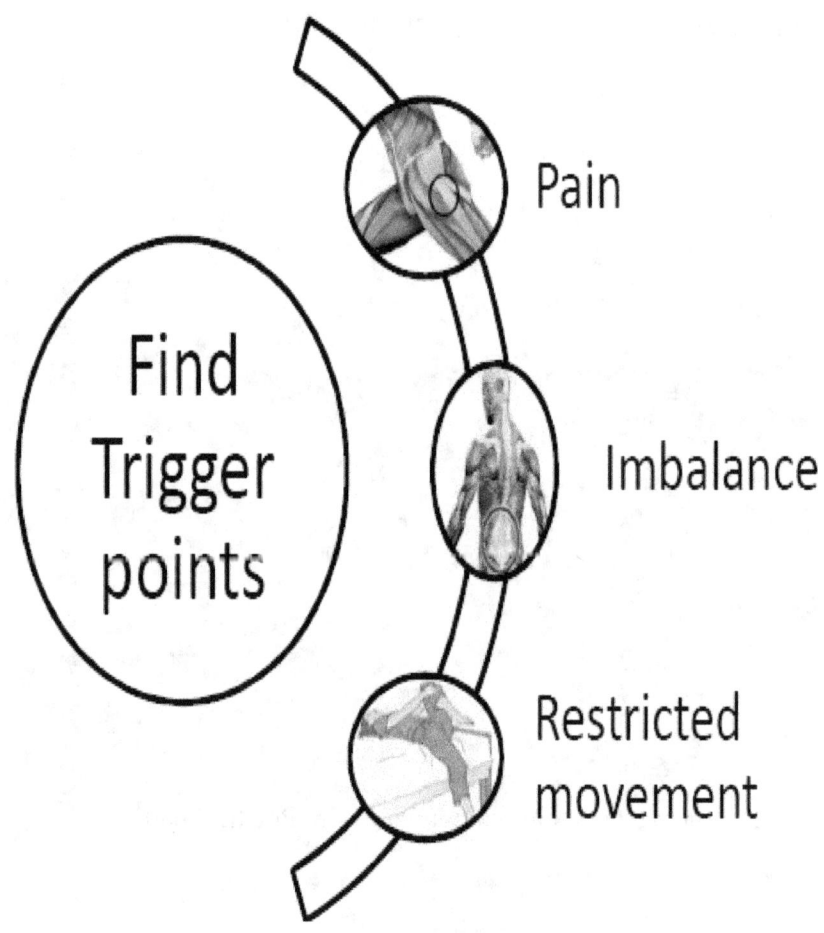

Whereas low level laser has many effects on fascia, this section is concerned with applications that lengthen shortened muscles, and normalize taut bands. This remedial science is known as MYOFASCIAL RELEASE

3.4 TRIGGER POINTS IN MYOFASCIAL DYSFUNCTION

A myo fascial trigger point is a point found in a nodule in a taut band of skeletal muscle tissue that is extremely tender and refers or radiates pain in a characteristic pattern. Trigger points are produced by muscle stress, such as overwork, repetitive motion, or sudden excessive stretch, surgery, strain, postural imbalances, and muscle loading.

The Physical therapist should apply knowledge of muscle anatomy in assessing the taut band, understand the specific muscles location and function. The motor or nerve sensory points fire pain on the taut band of shortened muscle. These points are trigger points. Treatment of the trigger point through laser may soften the taut band, increase muscle length and ease pain.

The process of normalizing the fascia and treatment of dysfunction involves identifying trigger points and applying laser treatment to improve the condition of soft tissue. This remedial therapy is known as Myofascial release.

3.5 MORE ON TRIGGER POINTS

Myofascial Trigger points (TPs) are reactive motor endplates located in skeletal muscle. They must be differentiated from AH SHI points, which will be discussed in the acupuncture section.

TPs are of different types. They may be active or passive, primary or secondary. All TPs are associated with dysfunction but only active TPs are associated with pain.

Primary or secondary TPs may be active or passive.
Myofascial TPs are generally specifically located in major muscles and classified according to clinical standards in this course. However they may occur in other places as the belly of the muscle, or near the insertion. They often occur near ligaments. A TP may maintain deep unpleasant aching, restrict movement and refer pain distally.

Dominating TPs may be difficult to locate when myofascial dysfunction and pain are more acute.

Active TPs are very tender on palpation. They may vary in irritability, and express various symptoms from time to time. The severity and extent of the referred pain depends on the irritability of the TP, not on its size, or on the size of its taut muscle. Active TPs may become passive after rest, treatment of precipitating factors, or treatment of the TP.

Passive (latent) TPs are less tender on palpation. They may be found in clinically normal patients and are associated with restricted movements and weakness/fatigue of affected muscles. Passive TPs can be activated easily by many factors, especially overuse/ overstretching, and can then trigger clinical pain or dysfunction. Fitter muscles resist activation of passive TPs.

Primary TPs arise as a direct result of physical injury, local irritation in virus diseases or direct environmental effects on myofascial tissue. Active primary TPs, causing pain and increasing muscle stress elsewhere, may initiate secondary TPs in the same or in other muscles.

Secondary TPs are those which arise due to foci of irritation elsewhere, such as visceral disease or as support to active primary TPs.

3.6 AETIOLOGY OF TPs

Normal fascia is not painful on palpation, and generally does not contain TP.

However foci of irritation may become TPs, including keloid scars, scar tissue, Sites of surgical incision, bruising, abscesses, local infection, vaccination or the like.

Fatigued, overloaded and undernourished muscles develop TPs during strain. Direct injury or trauma also causes myofascial dysfunction.
TPs can arrive during periods of rapid growth, or during infections, fevers and viral.

Internal organ pathologies give rise to TPS in muscles of nearby spinal segments. Arthritis, subluxion of the vertebrae, vertebral disc lesions or spinal nerve entrapment are also associated with TPs.

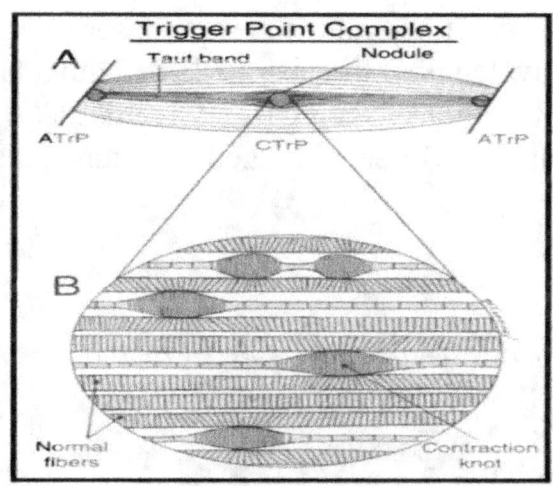

3.7 TREATMENT OF TPs

Assess the cause of the TP, the nature of pain, the quality of pain, the onset of pain and the duration of pain, what relieves the pain and the history of the dysfunction as noted by the patient.

TPs cause motor and sensory changes in the areas of dysfunction. Muscle coordination will show disturbance. There may be dizziness or other autonomic effects. Skin temperature changes may also exist. These symptoms should be evaluated.

TPs are removed by specific massage techniques, by laser or by injections. Positional release is also possible whereby the patient is positioned so that the muscle is shortened for some time in a rested state to effect a release.
This course is concerned with knowledge of TP locations of specific muscles as classified for Physical therapists. It has already been explained that other points may exist and must be identified that require laser application.
The laser dosimetry per trigger point is generally 2 to 6 Joules per point.

Sites of referred pain may be irradiated with laser. Generally one session should release the trigger point. Multiple sessions may be offered to improve the soft tissue condition.

Successful laser therapy outcomes, in particular with the treatment of muscle spasms, are technique driven. Poorly executed or improper methods can lead to less-than-desirable clinical outcomes. It begins with proper laser selection. An infrared (750 nm to 1000 nm wavelengths) therapeutic laser with a large peak power, or large energy density, without creating excessive tissue heating is ideal. CW lasers may heat tissue over prolonged exposure.

Editorial insights

On fascia. Super pulsed laser penetrates deep fascia. CW IR also does, but only if pressure is used to

A. come closer the target and

B. create an ischemic area, increasing the penetration.

For wounds: it could be added that distant areas of the wound (proximal) at advantage could be irradiated initially. This opens the blood supply to the wounded area, which is often obstructed by ruptured vessels.

As for WALT and other dosage recommendations: Yes, it is confusing, but they are mainly recommendations within a therapeutic window. Think "dose at target". Nothing written in stone.

3.8 PEAK AND OUTPUT

A super-pulsed laser will have a very large peak Power (greater than 15 W), but its average power Output is very low. Alternatively, a low-level or "Cold" continuous-wave laser may be used if the Mean output of power is less than or equal to 500 mw.

3.9 SCIENTIFIC APPROACHES TO DETECTING TRIGGER POINTS

Identification of the muscle spasm or trigger point can be done

1) Via palpation.
If there is radiating pain to a "referred" area with increasing over-
Pressure, this is considered a true trigger point
And one that should be included in the treatment Plan.
Standardized charts of location of trigger points in specific muscles may also be consulted.
The belly of the muscle and insertions are frequently tender and respond to laser.

2) The Impedance meter
A novel method of identifying and locating
Trigger or tender points involves the use of an
Impedance meter.

Since a trigger point demonstrates a decreased
Resistance to the flow of electrical current, it will
Register as an active point and be considered
A laser therapy target. Additionally, some laser
Therapy devices have attachable "photo probes"
Or light guides that can both assist with palpating
And pain rating of trigger points as well as provide
additional soft-tissue stimulation.

TP's may be several. Palpate and mark TP's. Some are active and some are latent. Treat each one till the muscle length returns to normal.

3.10 APPLICATION AND TECHNIQUES : PONTINEN's PRINCIPLE

Once a trigger is identified, it is crucial that the laser aperture be held perpendicular to the trigger point (target surface) with direct skin contact and

"Mild" overpressure. This facilitates deeper penetration of the laser and helps prevent reflection of laser energy off the skin surface.

Dr. Pekka Pöntinen recommends that the treatment of any trigger or tender points adhere to the following guidelines.

1. Identify and palpate trigger point and note
Pain threshold, pain level (on a scale of 1 to
10, 10 being the worst) and texture;

2. Laser the TP, static method, dose: super-
Pulsed lasers 1-2 J, continuous-wave lasers
8-10 J with mild overpressure;

3. Re-evaluate the TP and record any changes
In pain threshold, pain level (on a scale of 1
To 10, 10 being the worst) and texture;

4. If pain or spasm persists, reapply the treatment,
up to two additional applications.

3.11 TREATMENT PROTOCOLS

FDA requirement is that the Physical Therapist manages therapy in the applied framework of a treatment protocol.

It is necessary to maintain documented records of treatments covering:

1. Tissue condition
2. Principles applied
3. Laser specifications
4. Area of irradiation
5. Muscles in which trigger points are located
6. Before session and after session pain records using instruments or verbal scale
7. Joule dose applied per point.
8. Number of sessions.
9. Duration of treatment.
10. Rest time between sessions

Others records on range of movement before and after treatment of afflicted muscle, comfort level of the patient.
Clients name, age, lifestyle, gender, and medical history including drug history should be on record.

Aftercare, further referrals or drug interactions.

APPLYING PRINCIPLES OF ASSESSMENT AND CORRECTION BASED ON SPORTS THERAPY

Reciprocal Inhibition:

This is a physiological approach based on treatment of antagonist muscles in muscle cramps.

Reciprocal inhibition is used to treat muscle cramps. It is derived from a principle of physiology known as Sherrington's Law of Reciprocal Inhibition which states 'when a muscle receives a nerve impulse to contract, its antagonist receives simultaneously an impulse to relax.

The law of reciprocal innervation has described a reflex loop mediated by the muscle spindles. When functioning correctly the contraction of a muscle is supported by reciprocal inhibition of the opposing muscle. When malfunctioning, the reflex loop will cause compensation and poor muscle coordination.

In this system, a muscle sprain or cramp, will be treated through laser application on the antagonistic muscle. For instance a bicep in cramp, will be relieved by laser application on the triceps. Upon reassessment, the therapist can evaluate the progress and the need for further laser exposure on both muscle groups. This is likely to require one treatment only.

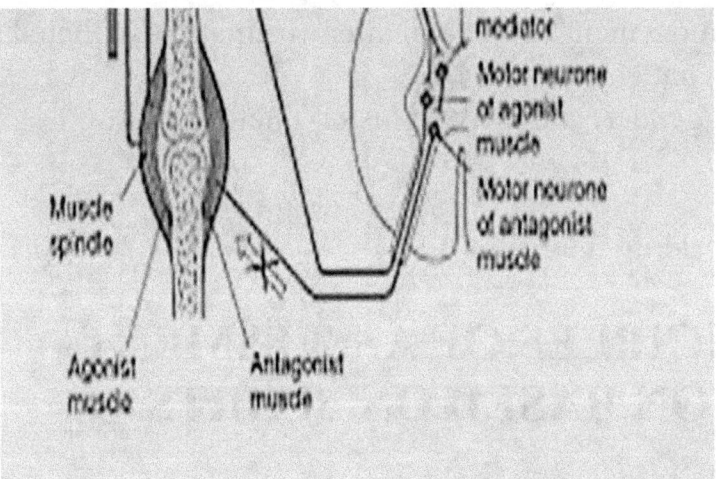

Assessment may be made through determining muscle functional balance and coordination. This technique is needed in advanced sports activity or post event.

Process:

Record a cramping muscle.
Locate the antagonist muscle.
Apply laser locally till the pin eases and the muscle relaxes.
Now again apply laser to the afflicted muscle directly
Whenever the agonist is much stronger than the antagonist, the agonist can overpower and injure the antagonist. This relationship is why most strength training programs revolve around balanced muscle pair exercises.

The following list comprises nine common agonist-antagonist muscle pairs that can assist a practitioner when using reciprocal inhibition techniques:

1. BICEPS – TRICEPS
2. DELTOIDS – LATISSIMUS DORSI
3. PECTORAL IS MAJOR – TRAPEZIUS/RHOMBOIDS
4. ILIOPSOAS – GLUTEUS MAXIMUS
5. QUADRICEPS – HAMSTRINGS
6. HIP ADDUCTOR – GLUTEUS MEDIUS
7. TIBIA LIS ANTERIOR – GASTROCNEMIUS
8. ANTERIOR DELTOID – LEVATOR SCAPULA
9. FOREARM FLEXORS – FOREARM EXTENSORS

Inhibition of the antagonistic muscles is not required for every muscular contraction. In fact, co-contraction can sometimes occur.

In the theory of reciprocal inhibition, reciprocal behaviours are defined as behaviours that compete against each other. For example, a relaxation behaviour in which the skeletal muscles are relaxed is considered reciprocal to a "fight or flight" stress response in which the muscles become tense. By repeatedly practicing the desired behaviour in the presence of the stimulus that used to trigger the undesired behaviour, the response to the stimulus is weakened and eventually, if the treatment is successful, the undesired behaviour is eliminated.

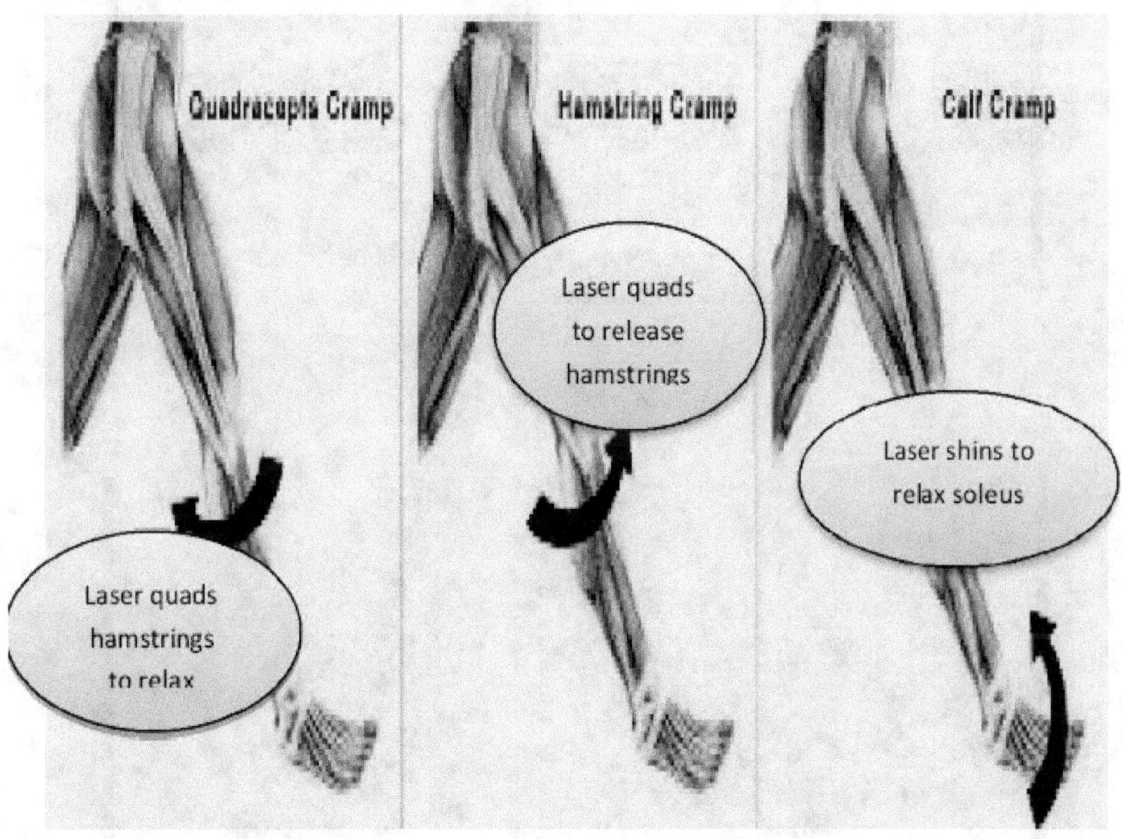

Positional Release

Many muscles require positional release to locate and treat TP'S. Positioning enables the therapist to treat hidden trigger points, that release shortened muscles and taut bands.

For therapy to be effective, the customer must be totally treated.
In the diagram below the upper picture is of positional release of the anterior deltoid, and the lower picture is of the posterior deltoid.

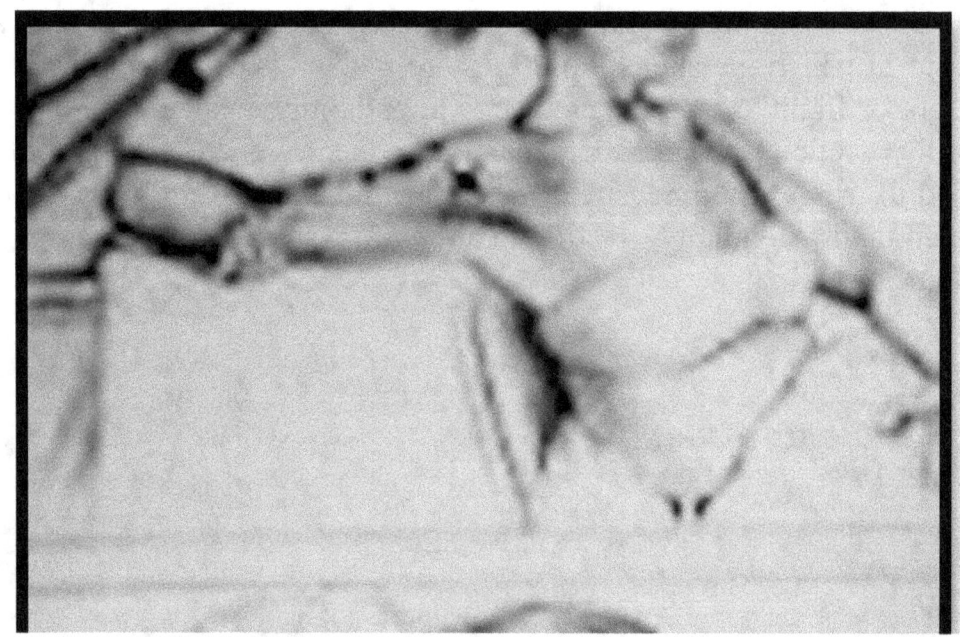

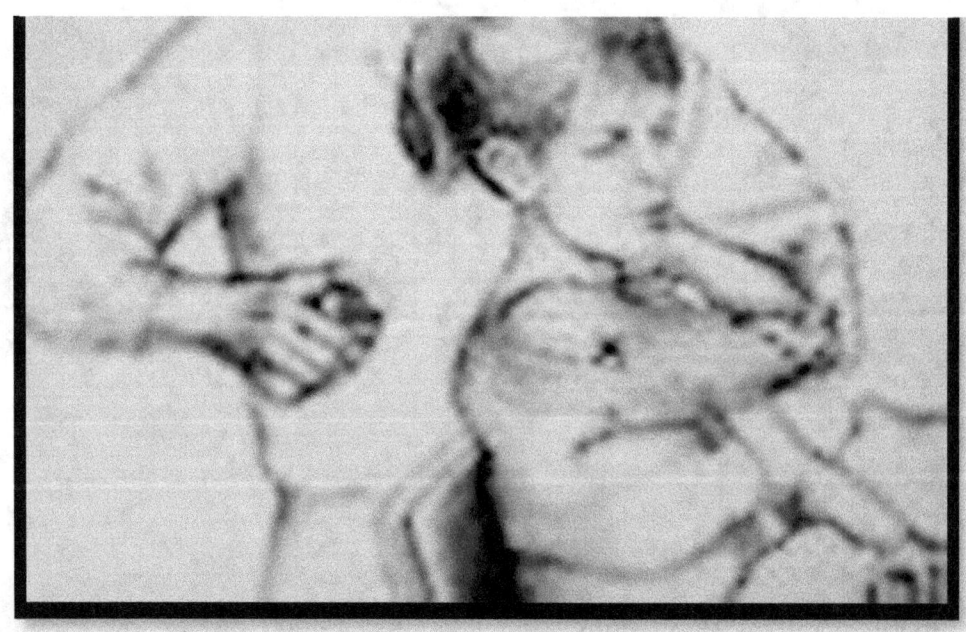

Positional release for Rhomboid muscles

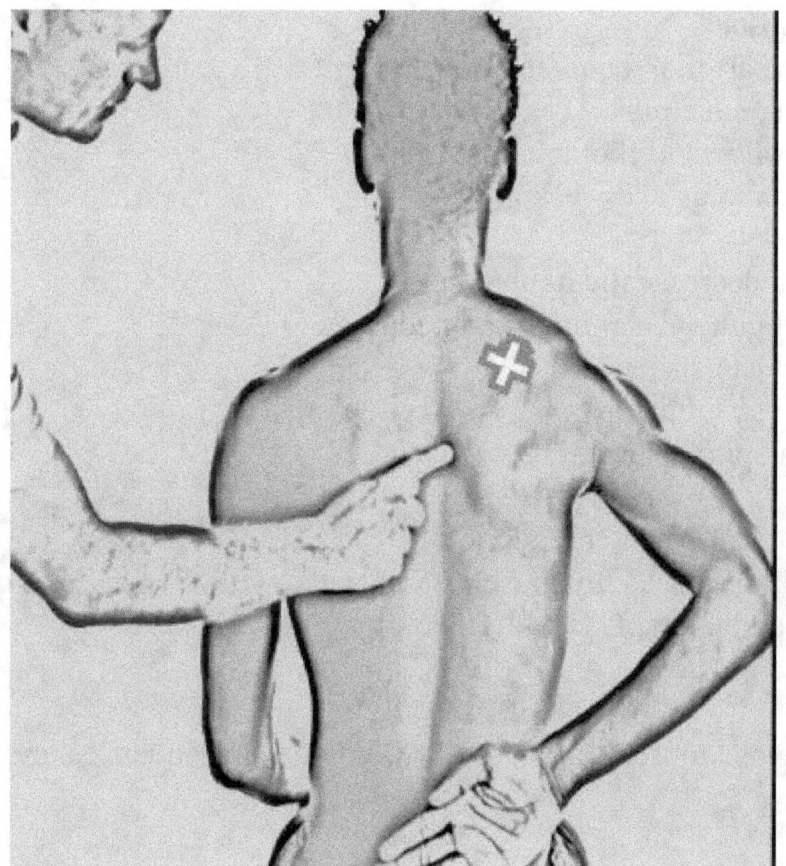

In the Spine, lumbo-pelvic balance must be assessed and managed.

Shortening causes curvature and degeneration of the disks. In this case the spine can be assessed and offending shortened muscles treated for TPs. Once they are lengthened, spinal flexion and performance and balance returns.

Whereas causes for dysfunction are numerous, LLLT TP therapy can be used to correct many deficiencies.

CHECKLIST OF POSTURE, PAIN, IMBALANCE, LIMITED ROM AND RELATED TRIGGER

Muscles that increase the lumbar curve and create an anterior pelvic tilt:
*Tight illliopsoas
*Tight/short sartoris, rectus femoris and TFL
*Tight/short adductors
*Tight/short fibers of thoracic longissimus.
*Weak abdominals and weak gluteals.

Muscles that decrease the lumbar curve
*Tight/short gluteus maximus and adductors
*Tight/short hamstrings
*Tight/short abdominals
*Weak para-spinal muscles

Muscles that cause a lateral pelvic tilt
*A pelvic tilt is caused my muscles associated with the pelvis as quadratus lumborum, adductors, ITB and TFL.

When shortened muscles are left untreated, the consequences are

*Postural imbalances
*Chronic pain,
*Compensation
*Poor gait and movement
*Weakens spinal cartilage
*Risks disk herniation

Therapist should manage detailed client SOAP sheets and assess risk of insufficient or delayed treatment, or related physical activities.
Positional release is managed so that the muscle is in a stretch which makes it possible to treat the TP. Deep muscles or underlying muscles are not

treatable without this stage of assessment and treatment. Some important charts are located below, as suggested by Travel and Simmons.

The key to treating TP's is to lengthen the muscle fibres that are short. As long as the muscle is affected it should not be loaded, jerked or forced. The therapist must tune in, and assess the depth and tension of the muscles barrier, which occurs at a very specific position.

The changes before and after treatment may be noted, as relaxation of taut bands, easing of pain, and more comfortable stretch or movement

Positional release for Upper trapezius fibers (below), middle trapezius and lower trapezius

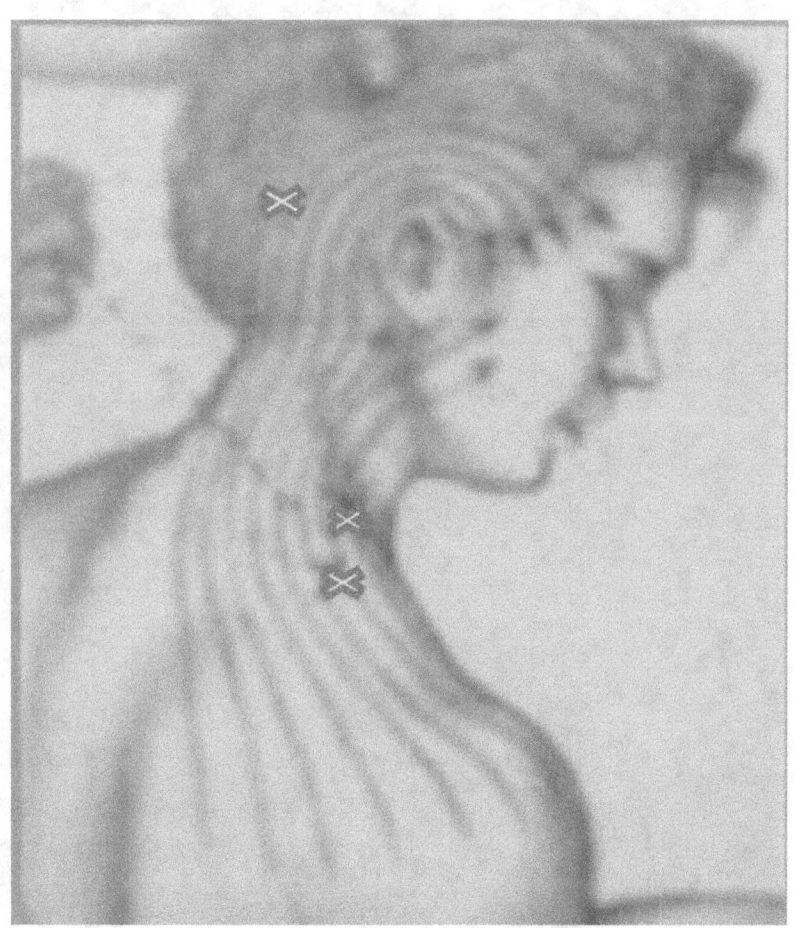

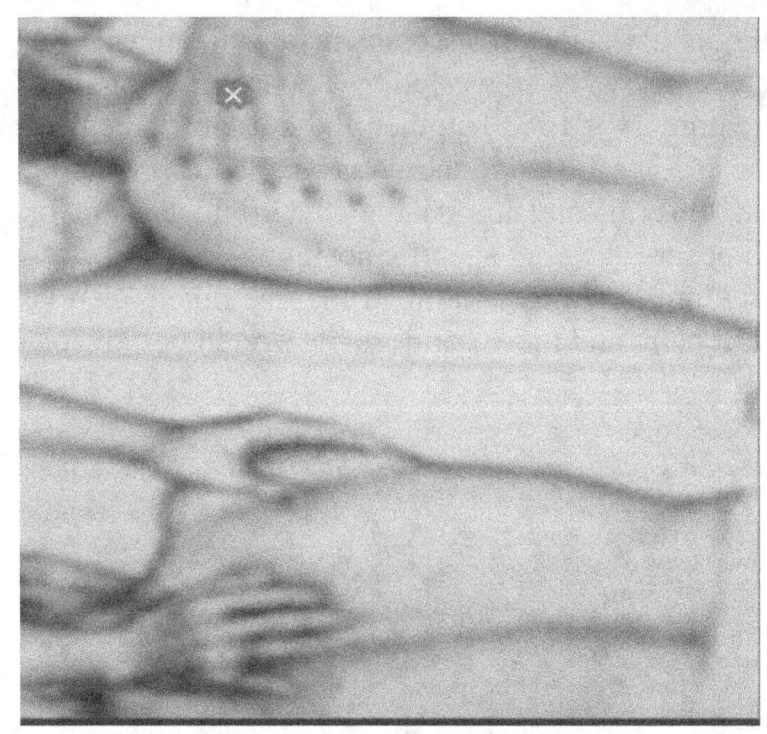

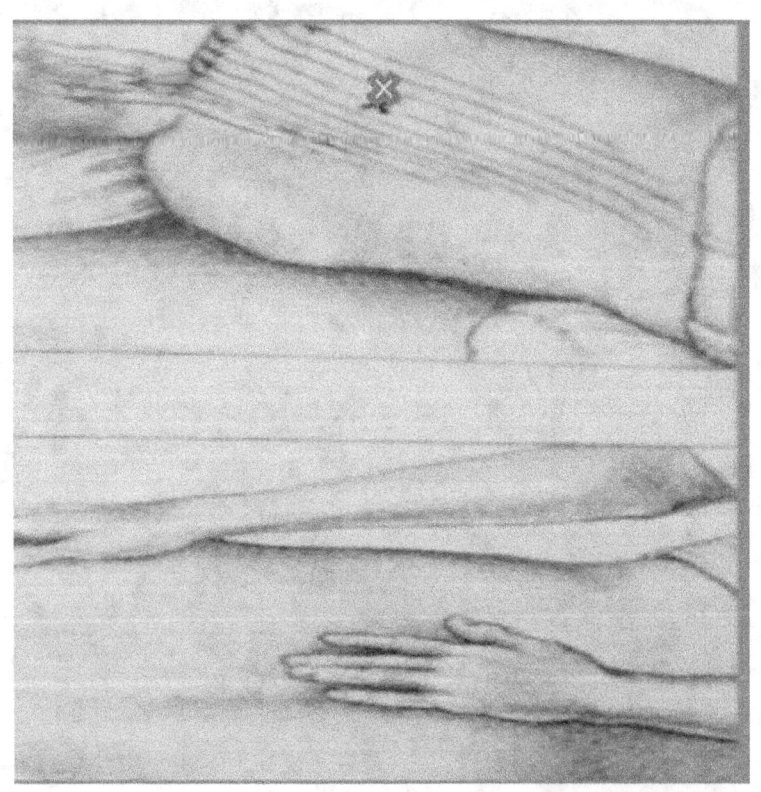

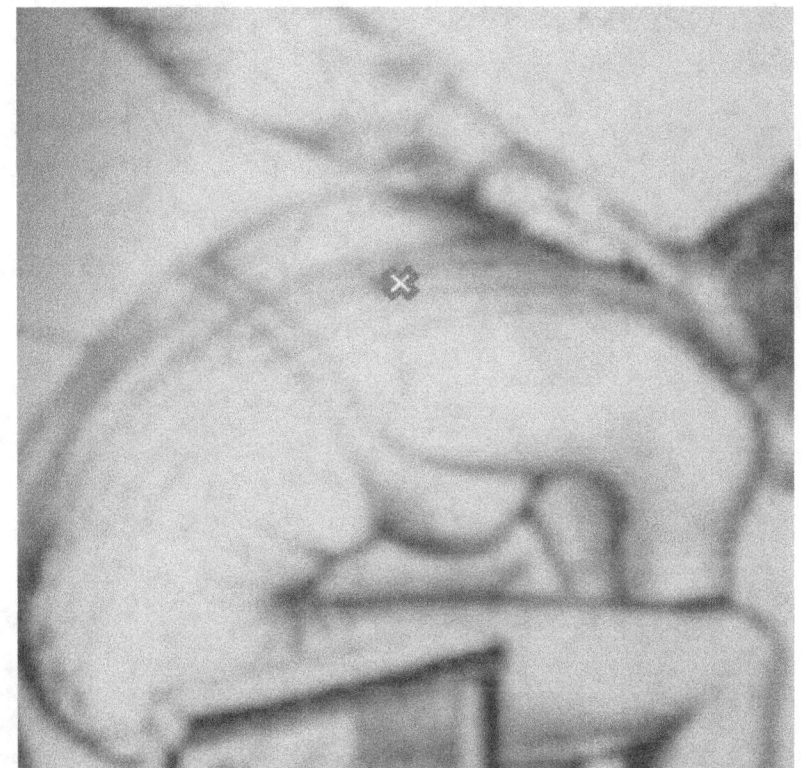

Spinal Rotators

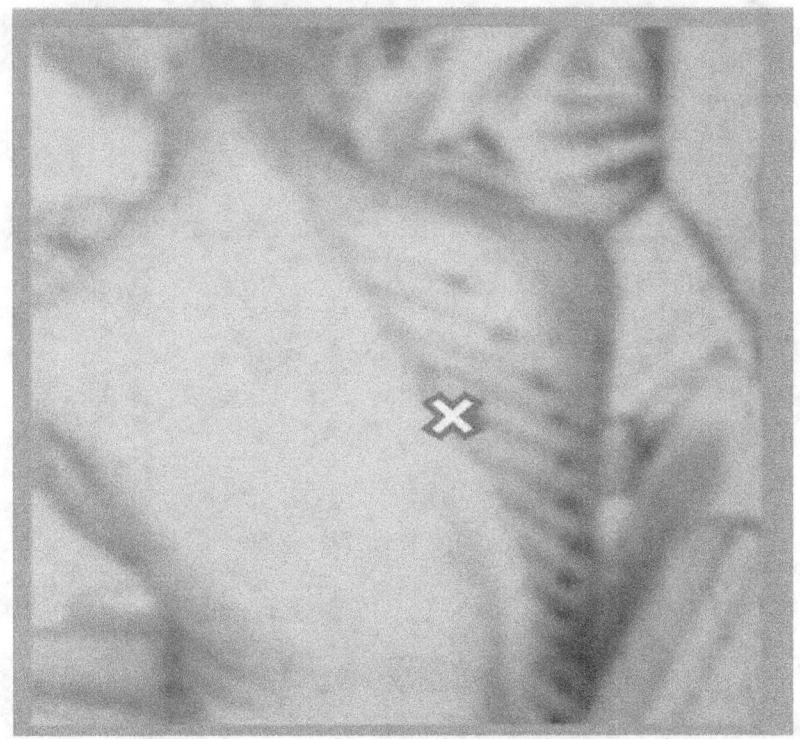

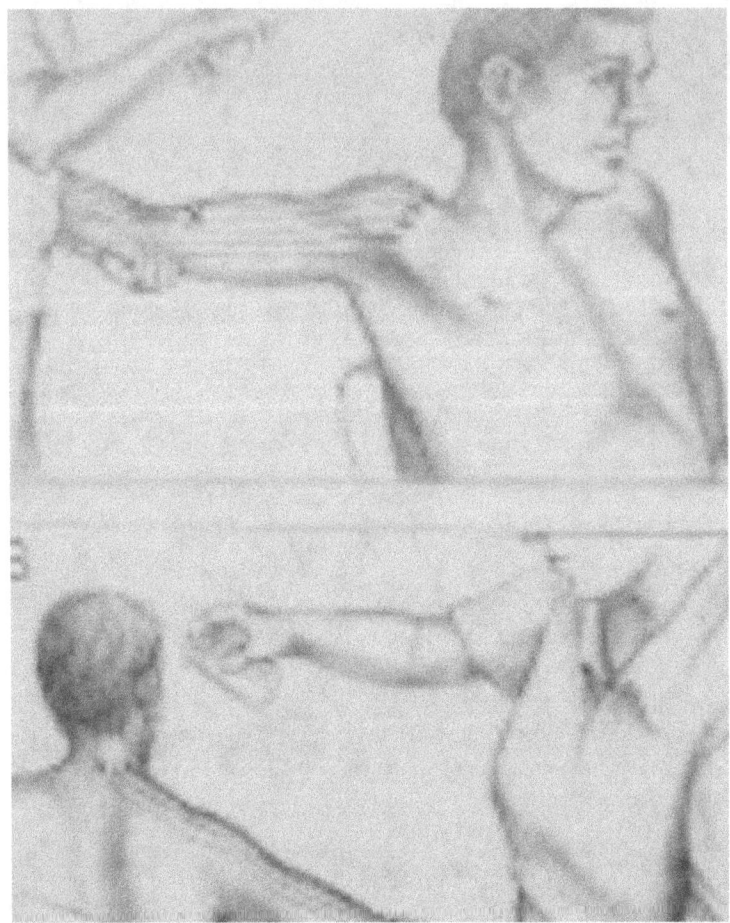

Positional release for biceps

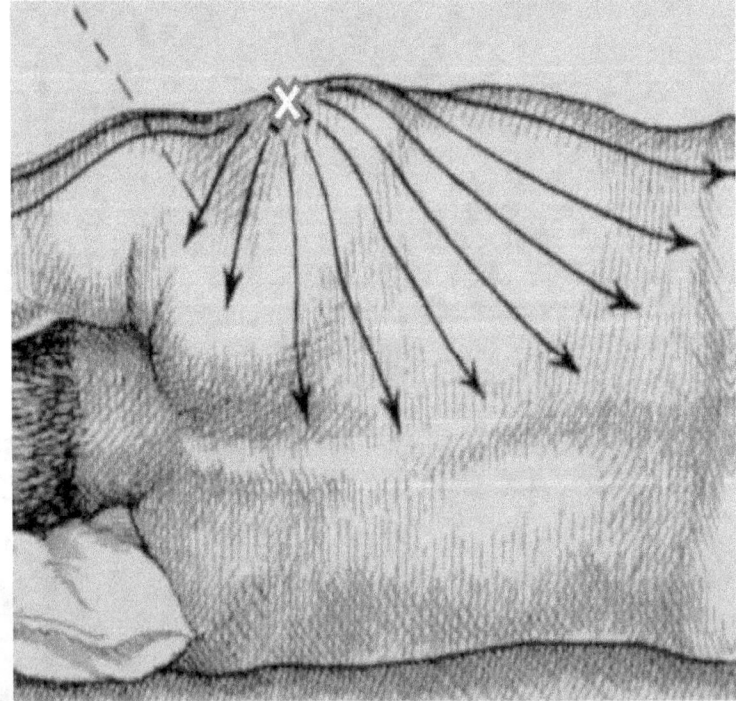

Position for release of latissmus dorsi.

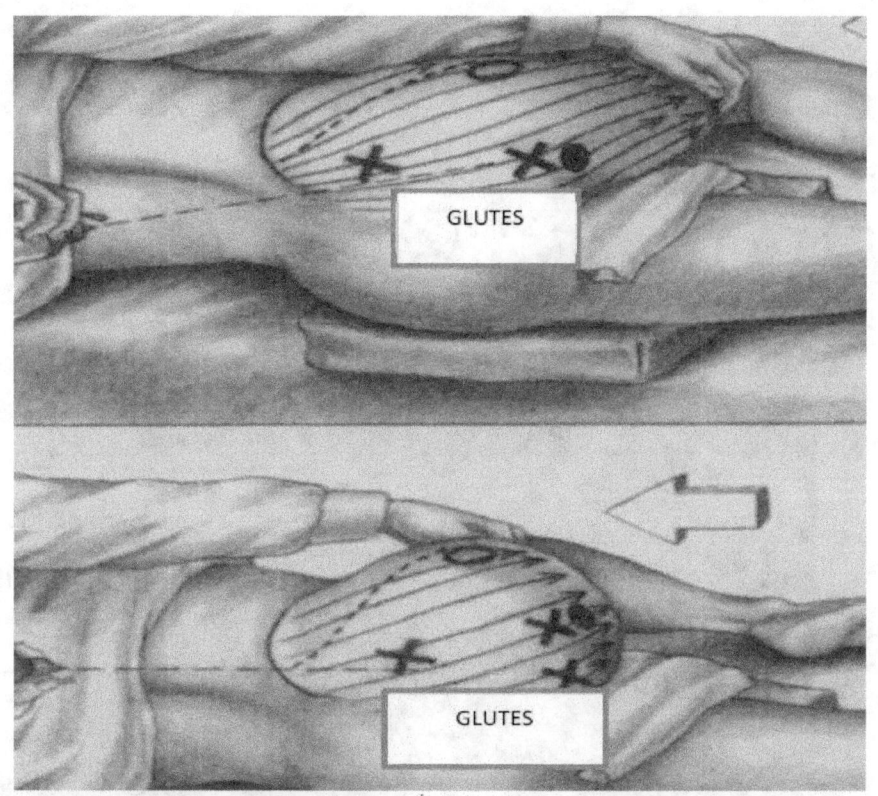

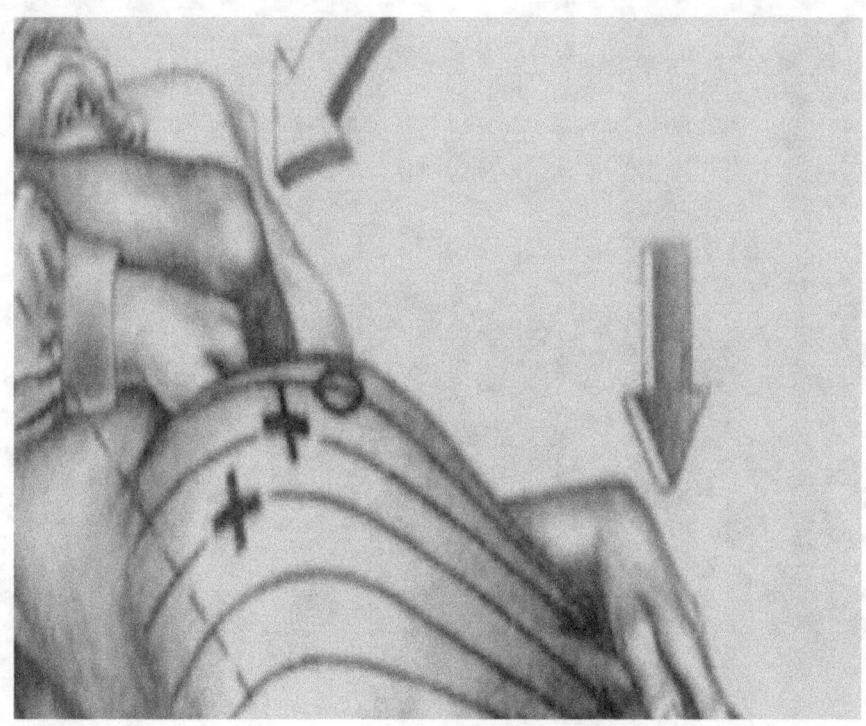

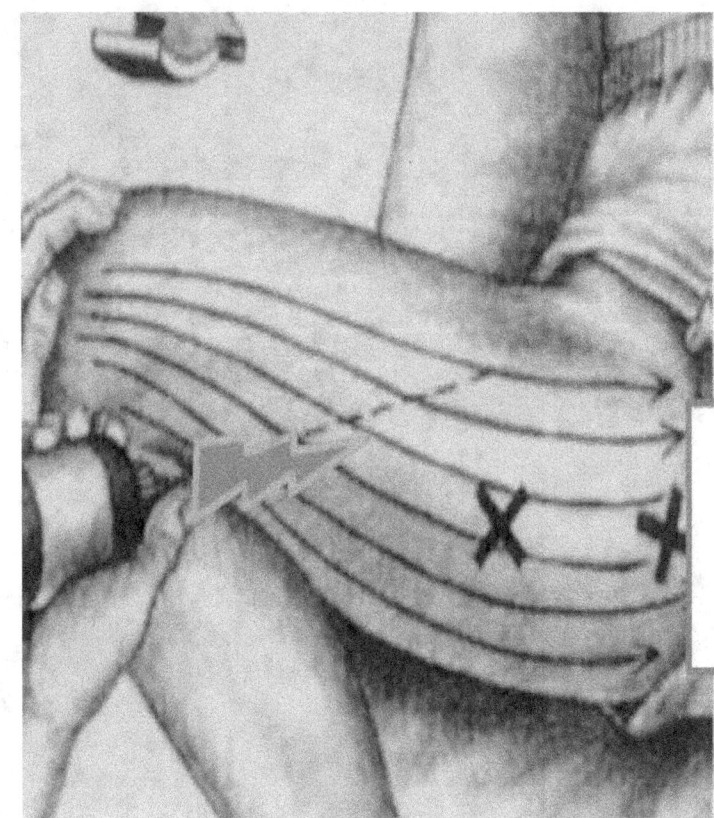

Adductor magnus, stretch position

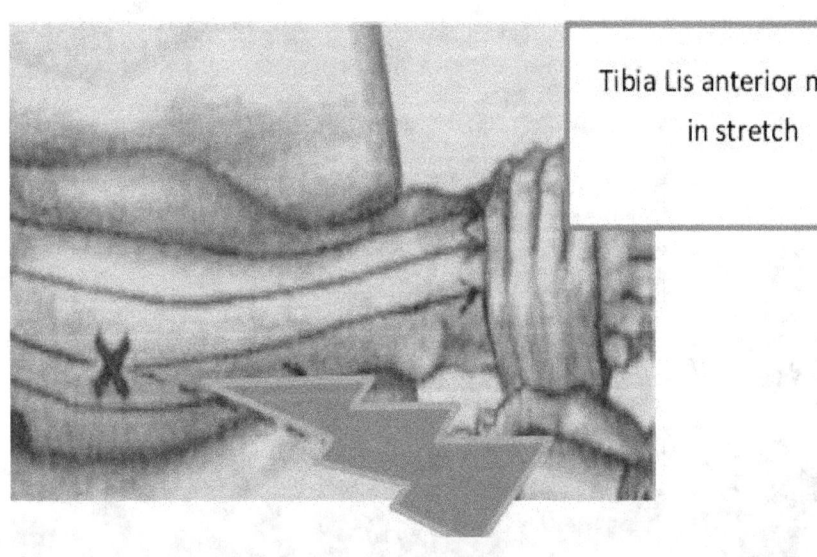

Tibia Lis anterior muscle in stretch

Trigger points and referred pain

Trigger Points refer pain to distal regions and the therapist must assess the origin of the pain.

LLLT may be applied directly on the TP and generally on the area of referred pain. Both places must be exposed to laser to regenerate damaged nerves and discomfort.

Vast us laterallis and pain referral

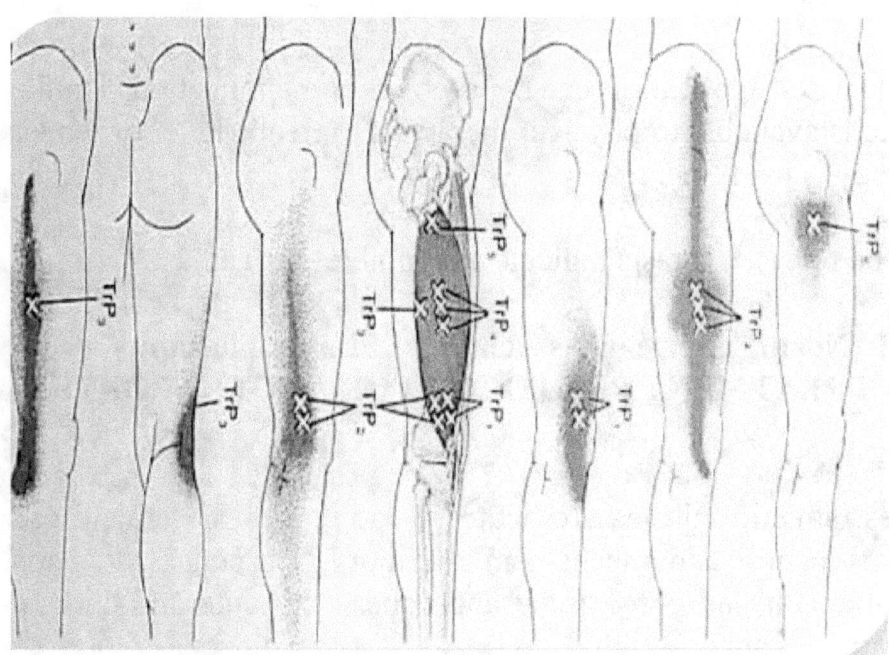

The records should be maintained to improve your own practice, and to reflect that you are acquiring the skill to treat maximally in minimum possible time. Your organization should have a policy of ensuring the security and confidentiality of records.

3.12 ON REASSESSMENT

Functional outcomes can be easily and objectively monitored via dynamometers, goniometers and dolorimeters to measure changes in strength, joint range of motion and pain thresholds following applications. Other tests may be applied for assessment to determine improved range of motion, strength and stamina, capacity to bear loads and counteract resistance, all indications of correct muscle function.

After a reduction of the trigger points, other modalities or procedures may be performed in the treatment plan. These can include soft-tissue mobilization, instrument-assisted soft-tissue mobilization, massage, traction, mobilization or therapeutic exercise.

The effects of the laser application can be seen in one application. Unlike many other methods available to physical therapists to treat trigger or tender points, laser therapy is pain free.

The patient may be released if tests indicate a complete recovery.

FROM NAALT (North American Association of Laser Therapy) MANAGING A TREATMENT PROTOCOL FOR ACUTE SPORTS INJURY

In most instances, athletic injuries are acute in nature and the athlete can describe the exact nature and mechanism of injury. Response to sports injuries can involve soft and bony tissue and consist of acute and chronic inflammatory healing factors.

Acute soft-tissue healing consists of the acute, repair and regeneration, and re-modelling phases. The acute phase lasts three to four days. During initial trauma, transitory vasoconstriction occurs, followed by vasodilatation and increased permeability. The second phase of soft tissue healing repair and regeneration extends from the inflammatory phase of 48 to 72 hours to approximately 5 weeks. It consists of resolution, development of granulation tissue, and finally regeneration of lost tissue, depending on the extent of the injury. The development of more granulation tissue in the second intention phase has a greater possibility of producing more scar tissue. Inflammation that lasts for a long period of time is termed chronic, lasting for months of even years. It may occur as a result of acute micro trauma and overuse. Scar tissue and degeneration are associated with chronic inflammation.

Applying laser

When electing phototherapy treatments for acute injuries, care needs to be taken in regarding what stage of healing the injury is in. Some phototherapy devices may emit a great deal of heat with the light, and this is contraindicated in the acute phase of healing. Clinicians need to be mindful of the stage of healing and to keep the "priority principle" in mind. Treating the injured tissues in order of significance is paramount to successful outcomes; these stages can be identified by the stage of healing the injury is in. It can be common for clinicians to focus on pain reduction as a primary goal; however, in the presence of acute swelling, pain relief would be secondary. While it is important to reduce pain, the first priority in these situations is to eliminate swelling to improve circulation to the area.

When treating the lymphatic system, it is necessary and prudent to treat proximal first, therefore opening and encouraging lymphatic flow from the distal area and to evacuate swelling at site.

As noted, treatment should begin at the most proximal site of drainage in the extremity. This is "Oshiro's Principle." The emitter should be applied with the "woodpecker" method-the probe does not move at the site; however, there is rhythmic pressure done to alternately compress and release the lymph vessels. Treatment should begin at the most proximal lymphatic vessel. Generally this will be located near the trunk-followed by any additional proximal sites to the injury. Upon completion of all treatment sites, direct treatment at the site of injury can be initiated. This will minimize the effects of lymphatic backup.

As the swelling decreases, proximal treatments will no longer be necessary and treatment can focus on tissue repair and pain reduction at target. The use of multi-probes and clusters to stimulate the lymph vessels is highly recommended. CW doses for laser (coherent) and LED/IRED (non-coherent) range from 8 to 12J/cm2respectively. The use of extremely high frequencies (1000 Hz to 3000 Hz) for 3 to 5 minutes produces better results with SP lasers.

In some instances, there will be increases in swelling during rehabilitation. Depending on the extent of the swelling, treatment may again need to target the lymphatic system. This may sometimes be the case when dealing with lower extremity injuries complicated by vascular insufficiencies. The treatment of tendons requires a technique that clinically has shown improved outcomes. Typically, probe placement is done at a 90-degree angle to the target.

Tendons, due to their dense composition and lack of pigmentation, are reflective, so to minimize reflection, the probe is held at a 45-degree angle to the tissue. Doses of 8Jj/cm2are most common for tendonitis.

CW lasers need to follow dosimetry value curves in order to achieve beneficial therapeutic effects. This means that the initial dosage may need to be adjusted according to the type of response the athlete had. A treatment response is a measurable goal indicating a positive result in the treatment of an injury/illness from exposure to phototherapy. A treatment reaction is an exacerbation of a condition/illness resulting from an overexposure of phototherapy. After treatment, the athlete's condition should be reassessed to determine whether there was a reaction, a response, or no response at all. If there was no response at all, dose should be increased by 2Joule increments at subsequent treatments until a treatment response or reaction is achieved.

A quick note about treating any type of chronic injury. Occasionally, pain can increase following the first few treatments, indicating that the light energy may have "pushed" the chronic condition into an acute phase of healing. This is not always seen as a treatment reaction; however, it may be necessary to decrease the dosage (by 2 Joules) to obtain the desired treatment response if the symptoms persist.

Treatment of tendonitis with a SP laser is slightly different than CW lasers. The aetiology of tendonitis is a combination of pain and inflammation. Therefore frequencies should specifically, address the tissue response desired. The application of the probe is similar to that of the CW setup; however, SP probes are typically scanned evenly along the tendon itself. The dosimetry is done again in unit time; however, treatments are done in "zones". That is, the same area may be treated with several different frequencies. The first zone setting should be set between 3000 Hz to 5000 Hz for inflammation for approximately 2-4 minutes. The second zone uses a pulse repetition frequency between 5 Hz and 100 Hz for pain relief. It is important to administer the higher frequency first. Because tendonitis can be chronic in nature and there is prevalent oral anti-inflammatory use, it is one of the more difficult conditions for which to achieve consistent results. It can take several applications before any results may be seen.

Other Considerations

There are several other considerations and recommendations that will help clinicians improve their overall outcomes with phototherapy. As cells and tissues recover, the need for continued stimulation by the device is lessened. So what may initially have been a stimulatory dose may eventually become an inhibitory one. A common mistake novice clinicians make is to increase the time exposure or joules. In effect, the tissue's need has lessened since healing and repair has occurred. The dose should decrease as time and treatment progresses.

It has been shown to be beneficial to treat at close intervals in the beginning (e.g., every other day or every third day for two weeks) and then at longer and longer intervals (e.g. Once a week for a few weeks). Experience shows that it is not disadvantageous to temporarily suspend treatment after a number of introductory sessions.

Certain considerations need to be taken into account when combining phototherapy with other physical agents. The use of heat or heating modalities should follow the application of phototherapy. The increase in blood circulation caused by heat may limit depth of penetration through increased absorption by haemoglobin at certain wavelengths. The use of ultrasound and laser has shown little benefit and may actually counteract each other. In the acute phase, heat is especially contraindicated. Some devices, in particular higher powered CW devices, can cause a great deal of superficial heat. Direct treatment to acute injuries may increase localized swelling and impact overall rehabilitation time. These devices can be used systemically (to produce a tertiary effect, such as lymphatic draining) and avoid direct treatment of acute injury sites.

A number of factors such as nutrition and blood supply can affect the healing process. A rule is that sports injury takes a little more than half the ordinary healing time if the healing process is stimulated with laser therapy. A common problem is that the subjective discomfort in the injured area soon disappears and the individual wants to return to training immediately.

It is essential that the injured are allowed to rest and that training be resumed gradually.

Treatment should not be interrupted just because pain is gone. This is only the first sign of recovery. Finally, return to activity should not be based on pain rather than function because laser modulates pain, but the healing may not have occurred. The modalities allow the athlete to regain the criteria for return, strength, and range of motion, more successfully. Several plateaus should be successfully completed before full return to activity is allowed. Patients are often so anxious to return to activity that they overdo, leading to a decrease in function with a rapid return to the results of inflammation. The goals of successful rehabilitation of overuse syndrome are pain-free range of motion, strength and endurance.

Phototherapy applications are helpful in meeting these goals in a shorter amount of time.

3.14 SOME GENERAL TREATMENT DOSAGE GUDELINES

Superficial fascia

Healing and pain management
Acute conditions 4 – 6J/sq. cm
Chronic conditions 6-10J/sq. cm
Open wounds 1 -2J/sq. cm (On the periphery to stimulate growth factor. Higher doses to stimulate wound closure.)
Closed wounds 2 -4 J/sq. cm
Manage to assess stage of wound healing, tissue condition, client type and other.

Deep fascia

Healing and pain management
Acute conditions 6 -10J/sq. cm
Chronic conditions 8 – 10J/sq. cm

Dark skins with more melanin will require larger doses as skin colour influences photon absorption
(For CW lasers) +2 J/sq. cm for darker skin

Body Mass should also be considered. Dense muscle and fatty mass requires larger doses than thin constitutions.
(For CW lasers)+2J/sq. cm for high muscle, adipose tissue. -2 J/sq.cm (from above recommendations)

3.15 OTHER GUIDELINES

-It may be more beneficial to treat small areas more intensively than to treat larger areas for equal time. Muscles with trigger points will have a protocol where the trigger point is treated intensively rather than the whole muscle. Anatomical concerns, tissue ionization and tissue adaptation are involved in the therapeutic response

-Small and more frequent doses are more effective than larger doses done less frequently
Treatments can be done daily two to three times

-Those with frail constitution, small children and patients with degenerative osteoarthritis, should be treated initially in small doses and graduated to a full dose.

-Acute conditions show results in 1 – 2 treatments

-Chronic conditions require 3 to 4 sessions before showing a therapeutic response.

3.16 ON TREATMENT OF TENDONS

Treating tendons is altogether a separate subject as medicine has very
Little means of healing tendon injuries.
Tendons require probes to be held at 45' angle to the tissue to reduce reflection.
This is due to the dense composition, lack of pigmentation and reflectivity.

The aetiology of tendonitis is a combination of pain and inflammation. Therefore application of specific frequencies should meet with the desired tissue response.

SP probes are scanned along the tendon evenly. Dosimetry in unit time is given in 'zones' – i.e. the same area may be treated with several different frequencies. In recent times the CW

Laser is preferred for the treatment of tendon for the benefits of higher accumulated doses and corresponding changes.

The first zone setting should be set between 3000Hz to 5000Hz (for inflammation)

For a few minutes. The second zone uses a pulse repetition frequency between 5Hz and 100Hz for pain relief. It is important to administer the higher frequency first.

A few applications are needed before results are seen. Generally the first five sessions treat inflammation and the next five sessions stimulate repair.

From Prof Pontinen

TREATING TENDINITIS:

Tendons are very slow to heal and rarely
Regain their original strength due to the rapid
Production of weaker, disorganized type III collagen.
A meta-analysis of low-level laser therapy
For tendinitis found optimal doses of super pulsed
Laser (905 nm) directly to the tendon insertions,
Seem to offer better short-term pain relief and
Less disability. Mid-range doses are required to
Stimulate the production of collagen.
From the author
Perform stress tests on the tendon and measure progress.
Ensure complete rest to the tendon during therapy phase. Exertion because
of immediate pain relief, can delay progress.

This author has successfully treated acute tendonitis in 6 to 8 session when using 904 nm cluster IR probes, combined with influential acupuncture points.

WALT 2010

Recommended treatment doses for Low Level Laser Therapy
Laser class 3 B, 780 - 860nm GaAlAs Lasers. Continuous or pulsed, mean output: 5 - 500mW
Irradiation times should range between 20 and 300 seconds
Diagnoses

Tendinopathies **Points or cm2 Joules 780 - 820nm Notes**
Carpal-tunnel 2-3 8 Minimum 4 Joules per point
Lateral epicondylitis 1-2 4 Maximum 100mW/cm2
Biceps humeri c.l. 1-2 6
Supraspinatus 2-3 8 Minimum 4 Joules per point
Infraspinatus 2-3 8 Minimum 4 Joules per point
Trochanter major 2-4 8
Patellar tendon 2-3 8
Tract. Iliotibialis 1-2 4 Maximum 100mW/cm2
Achilles tendon 2-3 8 Maximum 100mW/cm2
Plantar fasciitis 2-3 8 Minimum 4 Joules per point

Arthritis **Points or cm2 Joules**
Finger PIP or MCP 1-2 4
Wrist 2-4 8
Humeroradial joint 1-2 4
Elbow 2.4 8
Glen humeral joint 2-4 8 Minimum 4 Joules per point
Acromioclavicular 1-2 4
Temporomandibular 1-2 4
Cervical spine 4-12 16 Minimum 4 Joules per point
Lumbar spine 4-8 16 Minimum 4 Joules per point
Hip 2-4 12 Minimum 6 Joules per point
Knee medial 3-6 12 Minimum 4 Joules per point
Ankle 2-4 8

Daily treatment for 2 weeks or treatment every other day for 3-4 weeks is recommended.

Irradiation should cover most of the pathological tissue in the tendon/synovia.

Start with energy dose in table, then reduce by 30% when inflammation is under control.

Therapeutic dose windows typically range from +/- 50% of given values, and doses outside these windows are inappropriate and should not be considered as Low Level Laser Therapy.

Recommended doses are for white/Caucasian skin types based on results from clinical trials or extrapolation of study results with similar pathology and ultrasonography tissue measurements.

Disclaimer

The list may be subject to change at any time when more research trials are being published.

World Association of Laser Therapy is not responsible for the application of laser therapy in patients, which should be performed at the sole discretion and responsibility of the therapist.

Revised! April! 2010

Recommended treatment doses for Low Level Laser Therapy
Laser class 3B, 904 nm GA as Lasers
(Peak pulse output >1 Watt, mean output >5 mw and power density > 5mW/cm2)
Irradiation times should range between 30 and 600 seconds

Diagnoses Min. area/points Min. total dose
Carpal-tunnel 2-3 4 Minimum 2 Joules per point
Lateral epicondylitis 2-3 2 Maximum 100mW/cm2
Biceps humeri cap.long. 2-3 2
Supraspinatus 2-3 4 Minimum 2 Joules per point
Infraspinatus 2-3 4 Minimum 2 Joules per point
Trochanter major 2-3 2
Patellar tendon 2-3 2
Tract. Iliotibialis 2-3 2 Maximum 100mW/cm2

Achilles tendon 2-3 2 Maximum 100mW/cm2
Plantar fasciitis 2-3 4 Minimum 2 Joules per point
Arthritis **Points or cm2 Joules 904nm**
Finger PIP or MCP 1-2 1
Wrist 2-3 2
Humeroradial joint 2-3 2
Elbow 2-3 2
Glen humeral joint 2-3 2 Minimum 1 Joules per point
Acromioclavicular 2-3 2
Temporomandibular 2-3 2
Cervical spine 4 4 Minimum 1 Joules per point
Lumbar spine 4 4 Minimum 1 Joules per point
Hip 2 4 Minimum 2 Joules per point
Knee anteromedial 4-6 4 Minimum 1 Joules per point
Ankle 2-4 2

Revised! April! 2010!

Daily treatment for 2 weeks or treatment every other day for 3-4 weeks is recommended.
Irradiation should cover most of the pathological tissue in the tendon/synovia.
Start with energy dose in table, then reduce by 30% when inflammation is under control.
Therapeutic dose windows typically range from +/- 50% of given values, and doses outside these windows are inappropriate and should not be considered as Low Level Laser Therapy.

Recommended doses are for white/Caucasian skin types based on results from clinical trials or extrapolation of study results with similar pathology and ultrasonography tissue measurements.

Disclaimer
The list may be subject to change at any time when more research trials are being published.
World Association of Laser Therapy is not responsible for the application of laser therapy in patients, which should be performed at the sole discretion and responsibility of the therapist.

Below is another updated reference chart for dosimetry, based on stage of disease, recent, chronic or acute.

Clinical effect	Onset	Dosage level per point at start of treatment
Muscle tension relaxation	Immediate	2 J
Acupuncture point stimulation	Immediate	0,1 - 0,5 J
Nerve stimulation	Immediate	2 J
Release of contracture	Immediate/days	5 - 7 J
Improved micro-circulation	Minutes/hours	1 - 3 J
Anti-inflamatory effect in relation to acute inflammations	Minutes/hours	1 - 3 J
Anti-inflamatory effect in relation to chronic inflammations	Days/weeks	3 - 6 J
Pain relief	Minutes/hours	1 - 4 J
Revascularisation	Hours/days	2 - 3 J
Nerve cell regenaration	Days	2 J
Healing advancement	Days/weeks	1 - 4 J

Taken from: Clinical Laser Therapy

Note: Photos in this section of reciprocal inhibition, positional release and TP's are modified from Travell and Simons

3.17 SOAP FOR MYOFASCIAL DYSFUNCTION

STANDARDIZED CONSULTATION

Subjective, Objective, Assessment Plan

SAMPLE SOAP FORM.
Manage client intake, consent and records with great care

Create Highly Detailed SOAP Notes

This is a required skill for compliance in physical therapy to clinical processes and enables audit, or data for case referral to other units of physical therapy.

Highly detailed SOAPs can be written in seconds...
Every component of the SOAP note must be saved for that patient visit .
SOAP is Subjective, Objective, Assessment, Plan notes

Subjective

Introduction

The first part of the SOAP contains important information that the provider may want to know prior to treating the patient. Here mention reason for visit, appointment scheduling note, insurance case, appointment history, treatment plan and re-evaluation

Condition

The current condition case for the patient including the case name, primary diagnosis, start date and general notes.

List of Macros Include

Complaints, History of Present Illness, Follow up Visit Response to Care
Auto Accident Form, Personal Injury History, Visual Analog Pain Scale
Quadruple Visual Analog Pain Scale, Organ Non/Skeletal Complaint
Muscular Subjective-Upper & Lower, Extremity/Cervical Thoracic Spine
Dermatomes, Activities of Daily Living Affected, Outcome Assessment
Asymptomatic Wellness Visit, New Patient Health History
Review of Systems, New Patient Family Health History
Daily Habits, Improved Since Last Visit, Same Since Last Visit
Worse Since Last Visit, Naturopath, Personal Health History

Objective

Vitals

Quickly record height, weight, temperature, respirations, pulse oximetry, pulse and blood pressure within the system. BMI is automatically calculated, and even tells you if your patient is underweight, normal or overweight.

Free Text Objective Macros

• Vital Signs, Extremity Subluxations, Motion Palpation
• Palpable Pain, Quadruple Visual Analog Pain Scale
• Cerebellar Function Tests, Neurologic Tests
• Sensory Tests, Reflexes, Active/ passive Range of Motion
• Muscle Strength, Dermatomes, Orthopedic Tests
• Posture Evaluation, Lordosis/Scoliosis/Kyphosis
• Areas of Edema/Spasm/Tissue Changes, Palpation Findings/Thermal
• Muscle Tone Analysis, Activator Adjustments, Range of Motion Showing Improvement

Free Text Assessment Macros

List of Macros Included

Same/Better/Worse Tolerated Treatment Well
Patient States, Patient Compliance
Phase of Healing, Type of Care
Complicating Factors, Problem Category
Diagnosis Classification of Low Back Pain
Excused from Sports/P.E ADL's Showing Improvement
Range of Motion Showing Improvement, Cervical/Thoracic/ Upper Extremity
Muscle Groups Showing Improvement Lumbar/Sacral/Pelvic/Lower Extremity
Extremity Muscle Groups Affected Additional Lumbar/Sacral/Pelvic/Lower
Reflexes Showing Improvement. Additional Reflexes Affected
Absolute Contraindications. Maximum Medical Improvement
Recommended Patient Discharge. Excused From Work

PLAN

Treatment Plan

Part of treating a patient is developing a custom tailored treatment plan that makes sense for the clients condition.

List of Macros Included

Treatment Performed, Short Term Goals
Long Term Goals, Continue Current Treatment Plan
Additional Plan – Cryotherapy, Additional Plan – Heat
Stretching, Strengthening, Home Exercise Plan
Weight Loss Plan, RICE, Report of Findings Next Visit
Additional Diagnostic Testing Required, Referral
Sports/School Restrictions, Lifting (Weight) Restrictions

Malini Chaudhri

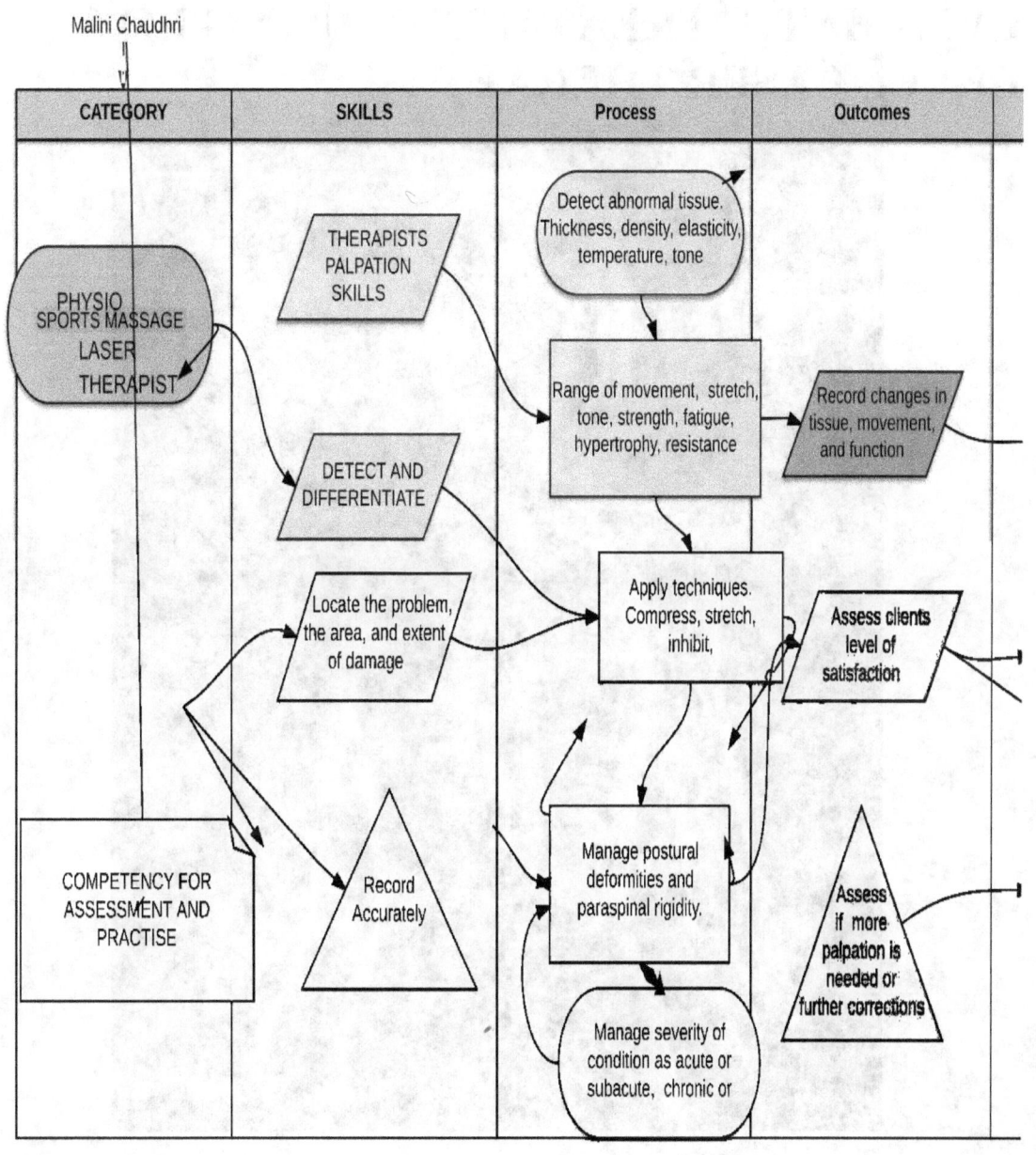

CATEGORY	SKILLS	Process	Outcomes

PHYSIO SPORTS MASSAGE LASER THERAPIST

THERAPISTS PALPATION SKILLS

Detect abnormal tissue. Thickness, density, elasticity, temperature, tone

Range of movement, stretch, tone, strength, fatigue, hypertrophy, resistance

Record changes in tissue, movement, and function

DETECT AND DIFFERENTIATE

Locate the problem, the area, and extent of damage

Apply techniques. Compress, stretch, inhibit,

Assess clients level of satisfaction

COMPETENCY FOR ASSESSMENT AND PRACTISE

Record Accurately

Manage postural deformities and paraspinal rigidity.

Assess if more palpation is needed or further corrections

Manage severity of condition as acute or subacute, chronic or

103

SECTION 4

LYMPHATIC TREATMENTS USING LOW LEVEL LASER THERAPY

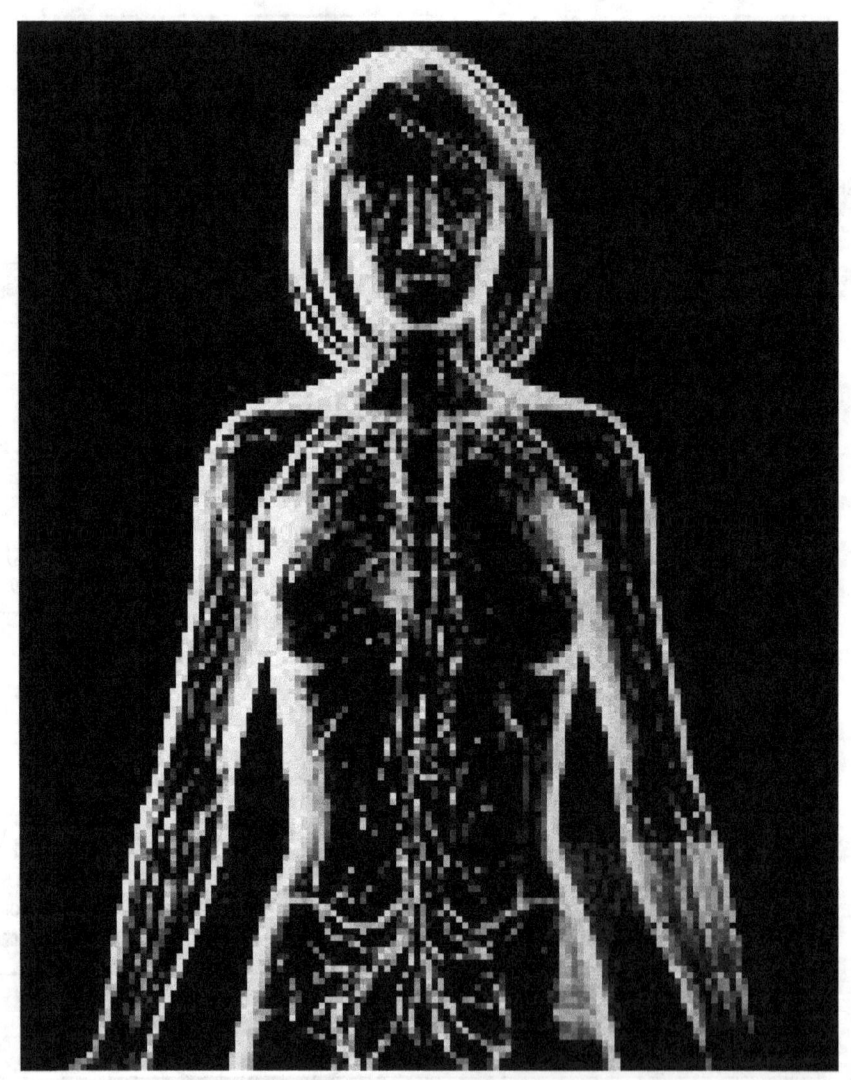

ANATOMY OF THE LYMPHATIC SYSTEM . LYMPHEDEMA
LOW LEVEL LASER THERAPY IN TREATING THE LYMPHATIC
SYSTEM

SKILLS DEVELOPMENT IN THIS SECTION

KNOWLEDGE OF LYPHEDEMA TISSUE CONDITIONS
PRINCIPLES OF LASER APPLICATION
TECHNIQUES OF LASER LYMPHATIC DRAINAGE
WALT DOSE RECOMMENDATIONS

CONTENTS

4.1 The Lymphatic System
4.2 Functions of the lymphatic system.
4.3 Disorder of the lymphatic system
4.4 Complications
4.5 Some Symptoms
4.6 Stages of lymphedema
4.7 Some basic facts about lymphedema
4.8 Laser interactions with edematic tissue
4.9 Treatment protocols
4.10 Some effects of laser therapy
4.11 Evolution of LLLT in the management of lymphedema
4.12 Reviewing WALT and AMLA standards
4.13 Acute Stage. Trauma induced
4.14 SOAP for Lymphatics

4.1 THE LYMPHATIC SYSTEM

The Lymphatic system is a relatively recent discovery in medicine. It is an extension of the Circulatory system. Lymphatic vessels and capillaries narrow down from the arteries to become a miniature transport system existing at the periphery of the skin. In a normal state the lymphatic move fluid to underlying and adjoining vessels and maintain the tone of the skin. Disease or injury may express in the lymphatic system causing toxicity, oedema and hardening of tissue.

The lymphatic system is a large system that moves fluid through ducts, vessels and thousands of bean shaped nodes in the body. The fluid is made up of water and proteins that feed the cells in the body. Lymph fluid is collected in the lymph vessels, filtered through the lymph nodes and it eventually drains into the bloodstream through large ducts in the chest (thoracic ducts).

The proteins are recycled or leave the body as waste in the urine.
The lymphatic system works with the lungs, muscles and the vascular system called the circulatory system. This is the system that pumps blood and supplies oxygen to the cells. The lungs and muscles are also important in moving lymph fluid through the body.

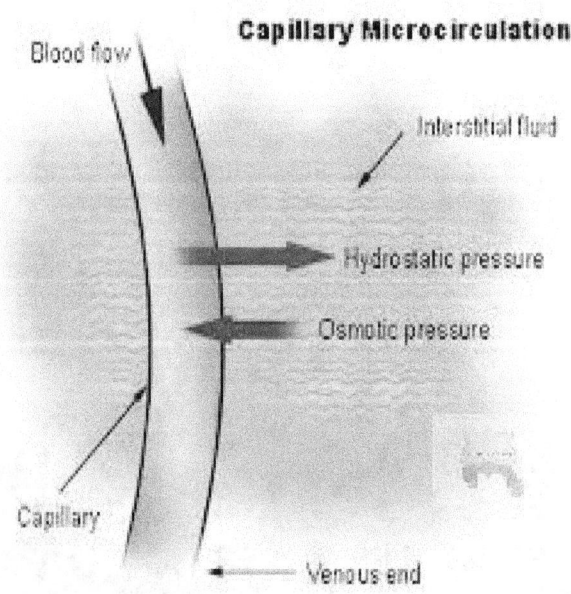

Capillary Microcirculation

Blood flow

Interstitial fluid

Hydrostatic pressure

Osmotic pressure

Capillary

Venous end

4.2 FUNCTIONS OF THE LYMPHATIC SYSTEM

The lymphatic system has two functions.

1) The main function is to help the circulatory system maintain a balance of fluid in the body. Fluids are needed to bring nutrients to, and remove waste products from cells. Every day about three litres of fluid is left behind in the tissue spaces of the body. The lymphatic system absorbs this fluid and returns it to the blood stream. This prevents swelling and balances the fluid in the body. Incredibly, the lymphatic system can handle up to ten times the normal amount of fluid in your body for a short period of time.

2) The other important function is to help defend the body from disease. When bacteria and viruses are detected in the fluid by the lymph node, it triggers special cells to remove them.This is why someone might feel some swollen nodes in the neck or armpit (Axillary) at times of infection or illness.

Diagram below shows the pathway of lymph vessels. Capillaries move from the circulatory

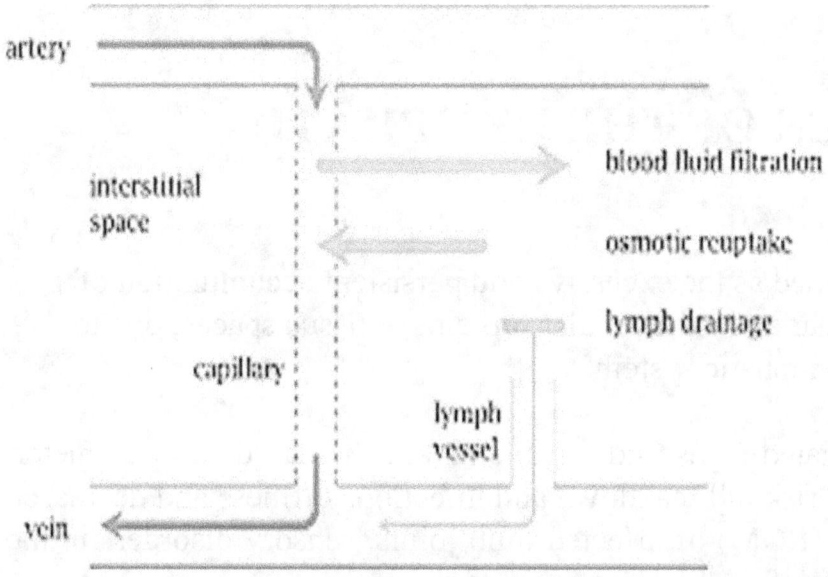

system, moderating waste proteins and cells through the thin permeable layers which are 1mm on the skins surface. Very light pressure moves the excess lymph towards the nodes where they are flushed out.

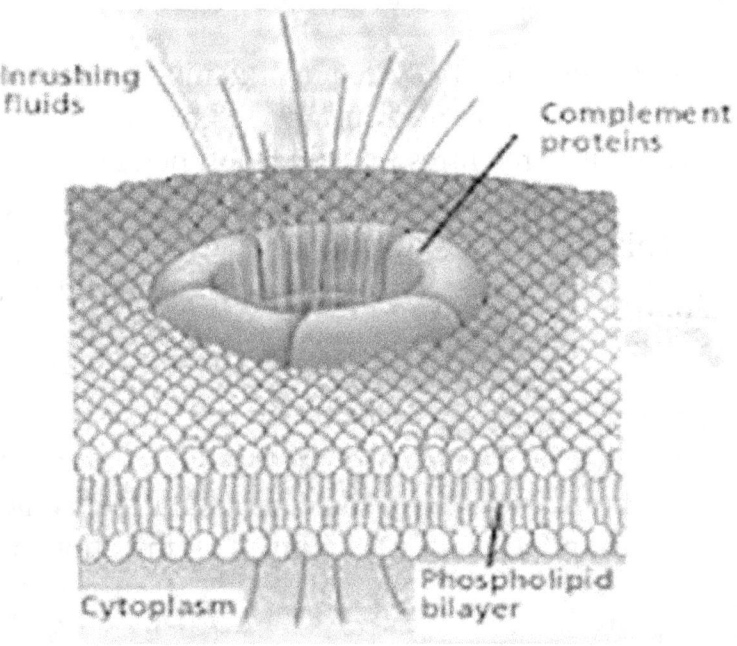

Strong pressure collapses the lymph, which may be caused by heart or kidney disorders, or through surgery.

4.3 DISORDER OF THE LYMPHATIC SYSTEM

Lymphedema is defined as the excessive and persistent accumulation of fluid and extravascular and extracellular proteins in tissue spaces, due to the inefficiency of the lymphatic system.

Lymphedema-associated signs and symptoms are increased limb diameter, skin tensioning with risk of breakdown and infection, stiffness and decreased range of movement (ROM) of affected limb joints, sensory disorders in the hand and reduced use of the limb for functional tasks.

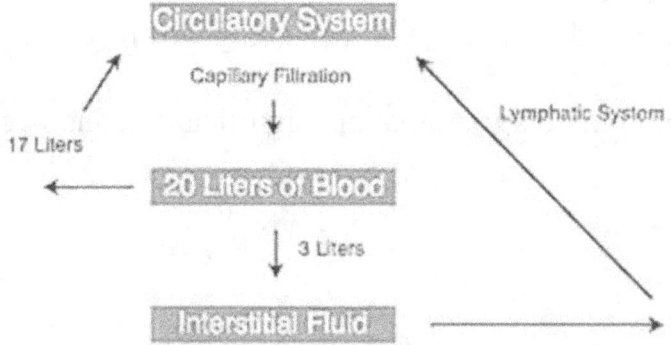

A single session of lymphatic drainage must move significant quantity of lymph in litres, and the results must be visible.

Lymph re-accumulates daily. Healthy lymphatic vessels and nodes move the lymph adequately. However during injury, or surgery, or cases of blocked nodes, the volume and static shift will show up. Low level laser can reconstruct lymphatic vessels, especially with 908 nm IR wavelengths.

ALARM POINTS: PATIENTS CONDITION

This disease can result in:

Aesthetic deformities,
Decreased functional ability,
Physical discomfort
Physiological and psychological stress

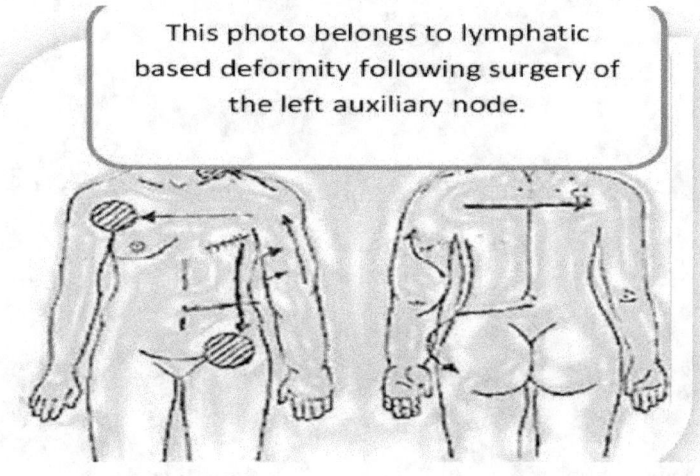

This photo belongs to lymphatic based deformity following surgery of the left auxiliary node.

Left untreated deformities increase and immunity weakens.

A check of important nodes and drainage is necessary to meet with therapies.

Important nodes are illustrated in the diagram that are significant in and neck region

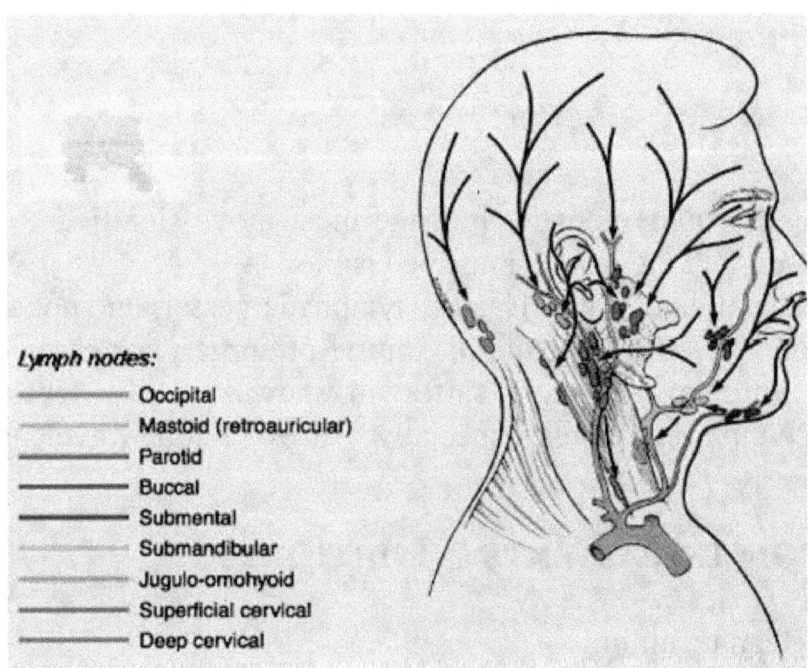

Lymph nodes:
———— Occipital
———— Mastoid (retroauricular)
———— Parotid
———— Buccal
———— Submental
———— Submandibular
———— Jugulo-omohyoid
———— Superficial cervical
———— Deep cervical

This diagram shows the deep and superficial flow of lymph internally and externally. The arrows indicate the direction that the probe may be applied in woodpecker technique. Over the valves the triangular technique may be applied. The face should show tone and reduced puffiness after the treatment.

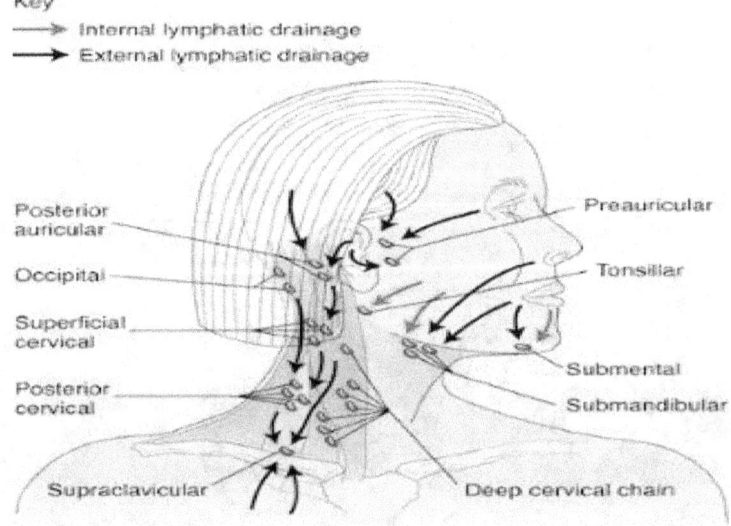

Key
——➤ Internal lymphatic drainage
——➤ External lymphatic drainage

Posterior auricular

Occipital

Superficial cervical

Posterior cervical

Supraclavicular

Preauricular

Tonsillar

Submental

Submandibular

Deep cervical chain

Other nodes in the body are observed in the diagram below Keep in mind that there is an invisible watershed. All lymph below the waste drains into the inguinal node. And all lymph

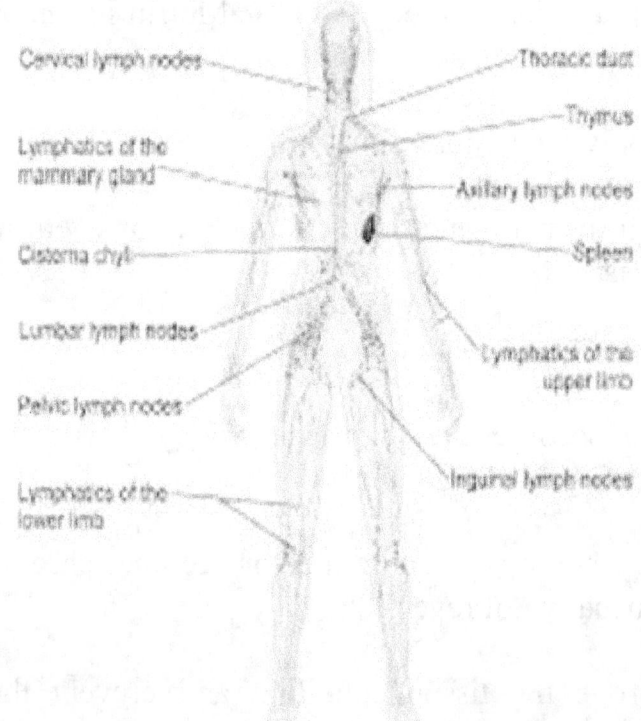

above the waist drain into the auxiliary node. In case one node is removed, the other node is able to filter, and lymph must be drained towards it. Laser probes must be managed skilfully with woodpecker technique towards the significant node in the area. Cluster lasers also support lymph drainage, in their capacity to break down hardened oedema tic tissues in progressed states.

4.4 COMPLICATIONS

Please have the oncologist assess the cause of lymph oedema prior to therapy.

Pain

This suggests a complication in the pathology. It is usually described as a deep, aching pain.

Often it will come before the appearance of visible swelling or an infection. Acetaminophen (e.g., Tylenol®) or ibuprofen (e.g. Advil®, Motrin®) can be used temporarily to reduce the pain.

Many patients report relief by applying compression.

Always record any signs of pain in managing dose parameters, or even, in referring the client to an oncologist.

Fibrosis:

Fibrosis happens when soft tissue becomes hard and feels woody. This is the result of dense scar tissue developing within the limb.

Lymphedema can cause fibrosis when it is left untreated or becomes chronic over a long period of time. It is usually not reversible.

Low level laser helps to improve the tissue condition and prevent the development of fibrosis.

Angiosarcoma of the skin:

Angiosarcoma of the skin is a very rare type of cancer that is associated with chronic lymphedema. Any open sores and purple Lumps (papules) in the swollen limb should be biopsied.

This condition must not be treated

Other complications involving blood clots, heart and liver disease, radiation, surgery or injury must be assessed.

4.5 SOME SYMPTOMS

Tightness in the rings on the fingers, bangles on wrists, in the chest area, around the neck or groin.
Infection of the lymphatics in the skin. This is called Cellulitis
Sudden swelling after an injury.

Sudden swelling after excessive physical exertion, or airplane travel;
Small blisters that appear on the skin of the affected area;
Fluid seeping through the skin;
Reduced, or loss of movement in the arm or leg;
In cases of mastectomy, lymphedema developing within 2 to 4 years causing aesthetic deformity.

4.6 STAGES OF LYMPHEDEMA

Clinical assessment of the stage to which lymph oedema has progressed to is based on the following.

Stage 0 a latent or subclinical condition where oedema is not visible despite impaired lymph transport. Stage 0 may exist months or years before overt oedema occurs

Stage 1 Early accumulation of fluid relatively high in protein content that subsides with limb elevation. Pitting may occur. Cell proliferation mat be seen.

Stage 2 Limb elevation alone rarely reduces tissue swelling, and pitting may or may not occur. Fibrosis develops.

Stage 3 Lymph static elephantiasis. Pitting is absent and trophic skin changes as acanthuses and warty overgrowths appear.

4.7 SOME BASIC FACTS ABOUT LYMPHEDEMA

Two types of lymphedema occur – primary and secondary.

Primary lymphedema is rare, and results from a congenital abnormality of the lymphatic system. Here the individual lacks adequate supply of lymphatic vessels.

Secondary lymphedema is the most common form and results from the interruption or obstruction of the lymphatic channels. Secondary lymphedema may be categorized as acute or chronic. Methods. This is the type that the Physical therapist must be competent to treat.

The chronic version is a more vexing condition, generally only minimally improved by technologies currently in use, with recurrence when therapy ceases. Most frequently, chronic lymphedema occurs post-mastectomy and following a variety of other surgical procedures that involve disruption of the lymphatic channels and nodes. It also occurs secondary to congestive heart failure, chronic liver disease, thrombophlebitis and gravitational dependency.

4.8 -LASER INTERACTIONS ON EDEMATIC TISSUE.

Enhancement of ATP
Stimulation of Vasodilatation
Reduction in Interkeukin-1
Stabilization of the Cellular Membrane
Acceleration of Leukocytic Activity
Increase Prostaglandin Synthesis
Enhanced Lymphocyte Response
Increased Angiogenesis
Temperature Modulation
Enhanced Superoxide Dismutase SOD levels.

4.9 TREATMENT PROTOCOLS

PRIMARY EDEMA –
Long term and comprehensive treatment with laser therapy as one of the treatment protocols.

Systemic laser treatment, irradiation of nodes and regional lymphatic vessels. 904nm laser.

This condition requires diagnosis through intensive medical investigation.

SECONDARY LYMPHEDEMA –

Patients have reported significant improvement within 1to 4 weeks of treatment, the maximum effects being noted in the first week.

Treatment may continually show improvement up to 12 weeks

Treatment protocol should ideally have an Intensive (and comprehensive) phase of therapy, followed by a maintenance phase to maintain results.
SP or longer wavelength CW laser are used at 1-4 J/sq. cm. For post mastectomy.

Secondary oedema, the axillary node is irradiated, along with the oedema tic upper limbs (FDA has approved laser therapy for post mastectomy lymphedema).

Oshiro's theory of Proximal Priority.
The woodpecker technique is employed for draining with laser in case of a single probe. This technique mildly pushes down into the epithelium to move the excess fluid and is lifted again.

Pressure should not be so hard as to collapse the lymphatics.

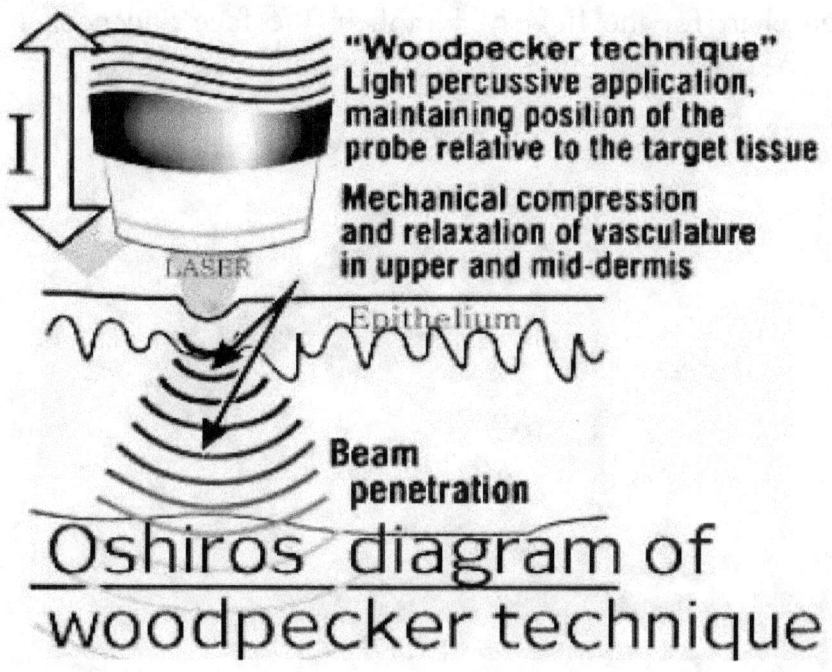

"Woodpecker technique"
Light percussive application, maintaining position of the probe relative to the target tissue

Mechanical compression and relaxation of vasculature in upper and mid-dermis

Oshiros diagram of woodpecker technique

Drain with laser probe in direction of arrows. Remember that there is a watershed, which indicates that all lymph below the waist is drained towards the inguinal nodes, and lymph above the waist will drain into the axilla.

Lymph is directed from the back towards the axilla and inguinal nodes

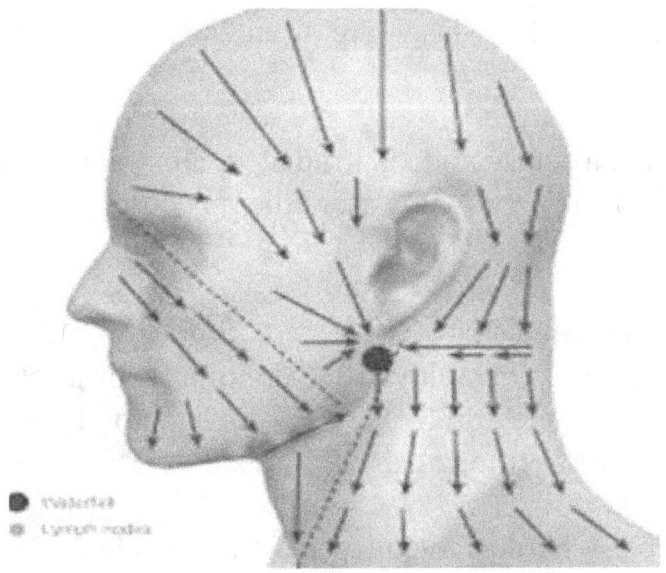

The face is drained in the direction of the waterfall- an imaginary demarcated chart for the flow of lymph in the face and neck region. The nodes must be opened and filtered with the triangular stroke.

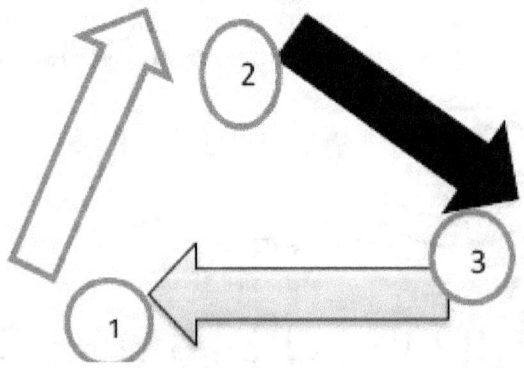

1. Push towards the draining area. 2-3 ounces of pressure

2. Move sideways from the draining area. 2-4 ounces of pressure
3. Pull away from the draining area. 1-3 ounces of pressure
Note that this is the exact pressure needed to open and close the valve and move the lymph through.

The node is filtered in half a centimetre diameter on the face and about an inch on the axilla.

4.10 SOME EFFECTS OF LASER THERAPY

Secondary Lymphedema reduction from laser therapy
Indicated the following hypotheses for its effects:
-restored axillary lymphatic drainage by the stimulation of new lymph conduits,
-softening of fibrous tissue and surgical scar,
-systemic effects related to the extracellular fluid volume and
-reduction of accumulated tissue fluids by blood flow changes.
Laser therapy also exerts analgesic effects.
-Putting it in practice still demands further research though.

4. 11 EVOLUTION OF LLLT IN THE MANAGEMENT OF LYMPHEDEMA

In 1917 Albert Einstein introduced the concept of stimulated emission from which the term. LASER (light amplification by the stimulated emission of light) was derived. In 1960the first Ruby laser was developed by Ted Haiman. It had a wavelength of 694nm and was soon used
for ophthalmology and dermatology.
Shortly after, in 1961, the first helium/neon (He-Ne) laser of 632nm was invented and became the first commercially available laser. Using this laser, Professor Endre Mester from Hungary became the pioneer of bio stimulation research at a cellular level. In the late 1970s interest grew in Italy, Japan, China, Russia and the UK, as technology advanced from expensive units
to smaller, more powerful semiconductors.

Research in LLLT has mainly centred on wound healing.

The use of LLLT in lymphedema management was pioneered in Australia in 1988 by Ann Thelander who based her work on Lievens' Studies of improved motor city of lymphatics and vascular tissue in wounds of mice. Lievens also determined microscopically that LLLT had a dilatory effect on those lymphatics in which oedema had been artificially induced, but had little or no effect on vessels not subjected to trauma of lymphatics and vascular tissue in wounds of mice. Lievens also determined microscopically that LLLT had a dilatory effect on those lymphatics in which oedema had been artificially induced, but had little or no effect on vessels
not subjected to trauma.

4.12 REVIEWING WALT AND AMLA STANDARDS

Literature available has a wide variety of treatment methods based on dosage, number of points, use of scanners or hand held probes, duration of therapy and use of combination probes. Lymph oedema does not have a precise standard for treatment.

Complications also exist based on Body mass index, the degree of fibrosis, initial ECV values and progression of disease.

Despite the need for more research on the subject WALT and AMLA have announced some dosages for successful therapy in post mastectomy lymph oedema. These prescriptions are currently the most likely to be used by therapists for predictable outcomes from therapy.

Diagram of a node

Diagram of a Lymph Node

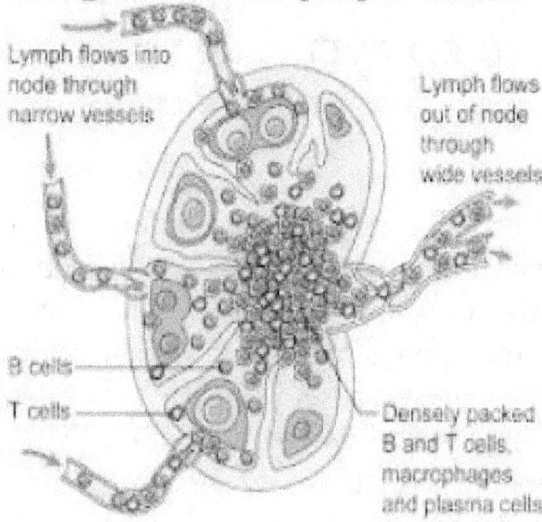

Lymph flows into node through narrow vessels

Lymph flows out of node through wide vessels

B cells

T cells

Densely packed B and T cells, macrophages and plasma cells

Diagram of a node

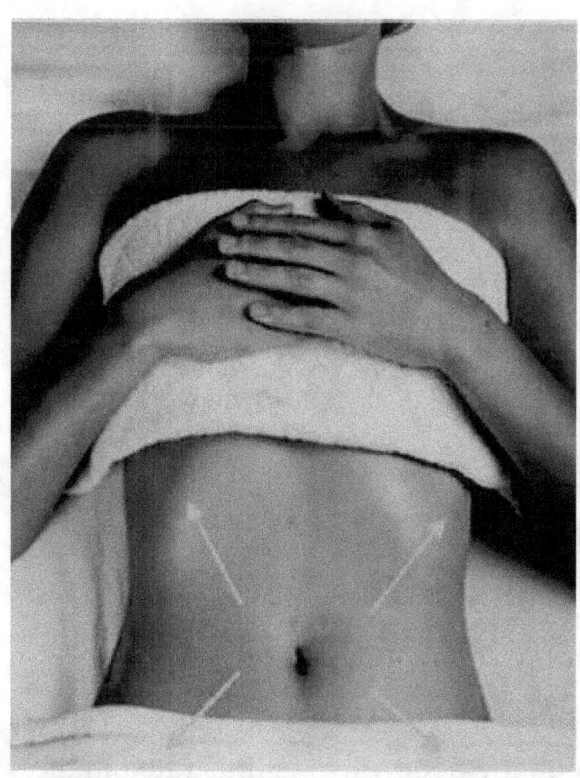

Follow directions of arrows for drainage directions of abdomen.

CLINICAL PRACTICE: DEVELOPMENT

Area of treatment

Proximal nodes and vessels are irradiated before any distal areas (I.e. axilla in the case of upper limbs and groin for lower limbs) to stimulate the dilatory effect and flow proximally as with manual lymph drainage techniques. Direct irradiation is often performed over areas of fibrosis.

In the case of scanning lasers, it is common practice in Australia to treat four to five areas of proximal to distal progression. The hand-held units are used directly over fibrotic or congested areas at a dose of 1.5j/sq. cm2 (equivalent to one minute of irradiation) per point.

Anatomy of a valve in the node.

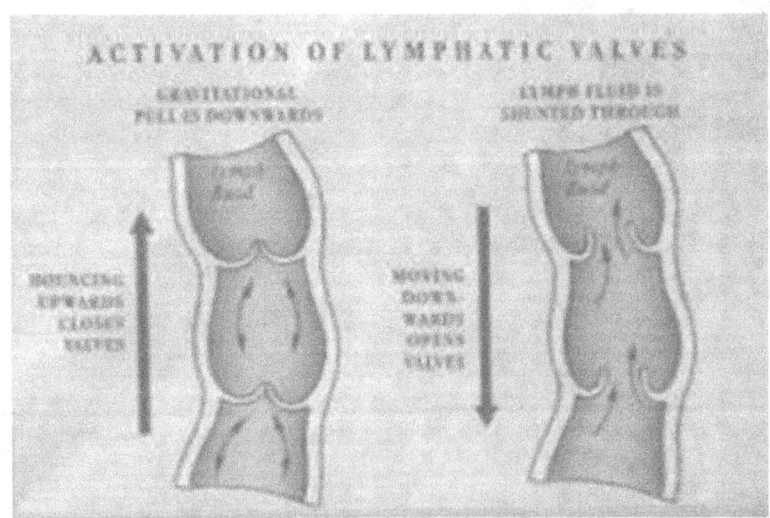

MOVING UPWARDS CLOSES VALVES
MOVING DOWNWARDS OPENS VALVES

The technique of draining lymph through the node valve is illustrated in the diagrams above.

Whereas woodpecker stroke moves the lymph flow in a specific direction towards the ducts, the triangular 3 step process over the submandibular, cervical and axillary nodes moves the lymph through the semi permeable membrane. In this stroke the node valve is opened, shifted and closed again.

Dose

As previously discussed, the therapeutic window is 0.5–4j/cm2 per treatment area. Doses too high can be bio-inhibitory.

The majority of studies researching lymph oedema have used 1.5j/cm2 in Spot application of up to 20 areas.

Scanning lasers likewise treat multiple areas with energy densities generally between 0.5– 2j/cm2. Hence, the cumulative dose in one session could be up to 20–30j/cm2.

Drain into axilla, the main lymph ducts of the upper body from all sides to start and conclude upper body laser lymphatic drainage treatments.
Use the three step triangular stroke over the axilla lymph valve to fully drain out.

For face lymph drainage, follow the direction of all arrows with a laser probe using woodpecker technique and move into the cervical node. Over the node valve, apply the three step triangular movement with a laser probe for long term procedure. Failing to complete the final step creates only a temporary situation.

Treatment Frequency

Research indicates that due to a cumulative effect over several sessions, the frequency of treatments can be reduced while still achieving or maintaining positive results.

In the studies discussed, treatment frequency was three times per week for several weeks at a time (interspersed with a block of no treatment), with up to 18 sessions in total over three to four months.

4.12 EARLY STAGE

Mild swelling and irregularities on one side that is noticeable and causes discomfort may be managed with Low level laser irradiation. Direct exposure improves the drainage, circulation, inflammation and removal of toxic waste.

Pictures show a foot that is reflecting the early onset of oedema. The second photo shows the direction for drainage with a probe to reduce the swelling. Note the crease on the rings of the left toes.

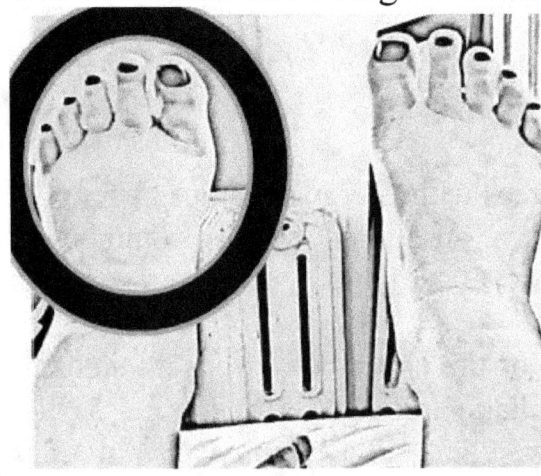

Lymphatic drainage of the foot. Follow directions of arrows.

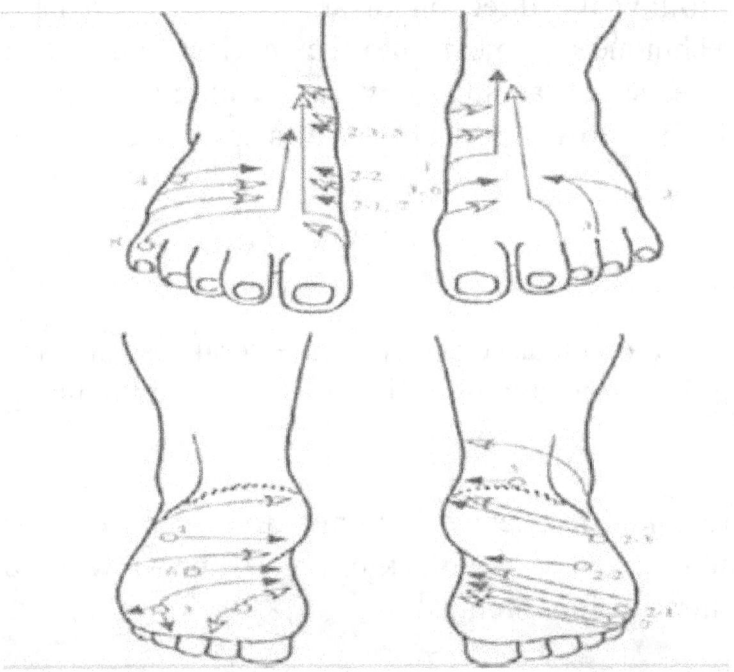

Anatomical correspondences to lymphatics on foot.

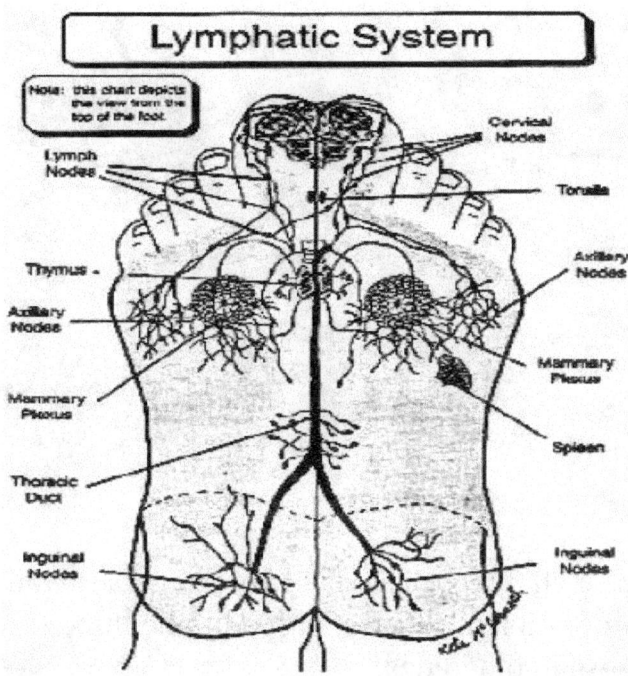

From reflexologyinstitute.com

4.13 ACUTE STAGE – TRAUMA INDUCED

Physical therapists often have to develop treatment protocols which consider and prioritize the presence of oedema tic tissue when treating a musculo-skeletal, or sports injury.

OSHIRO's PRIORITY PRINCIPLE is of utmost importance in the treatment of oedema or inflammation.

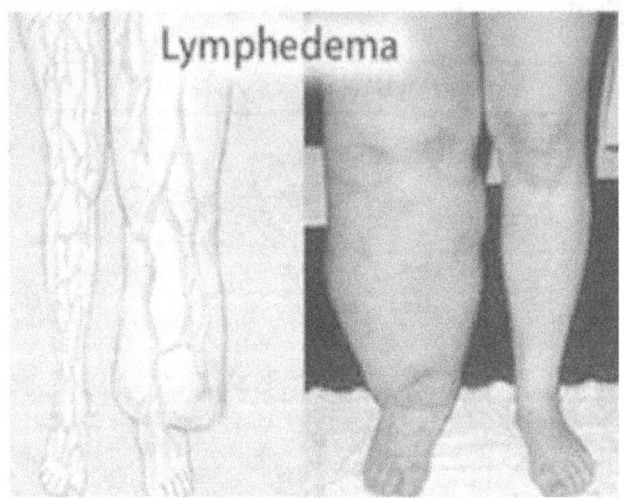

This states that care should be taken of the stage of healing. Treating the injured tissue in order of significance, based on the three stages of healing, is paramount to successful outcomes.

Clinicians generally focus on pain reduction as the primary goal. However, in the presence of acute swelling, pain relief should be secondary. The first priority would be to decrease swelling to improve circulation in the area.
Lymphatic drainage is facilitated by treating proximal areas to the injury, thereby opening and encouraging lymphatic flow from the distal area and evacuating swelling at the site.

A 'woodpecker' method of contact with the probe enhances lymphatic flow, as there is a rhythmic pressure to compress and release the lymph vessels.
(In the presence of oedema, immediate pain reduction treatments can increase swelling and block drainage)Upon completion of proximal treatment sites, direct treatment of the injury can be initiated. Swelling will be under control and the effects of lymphatic back up will be reduced.

Once swelling has been reduced it is not necessary to continue treatment of oedema.

The use of cluster probes to stimulate the lymph vessels is highly recommended.

CW doses for lymphatic drainage range from 8 – 12 J/sq. cm
SP lasers show results with high frequencies (1000 Hz to 3000 Hz)

Drainage is always a very mild stroke using minimum pressure with the laser

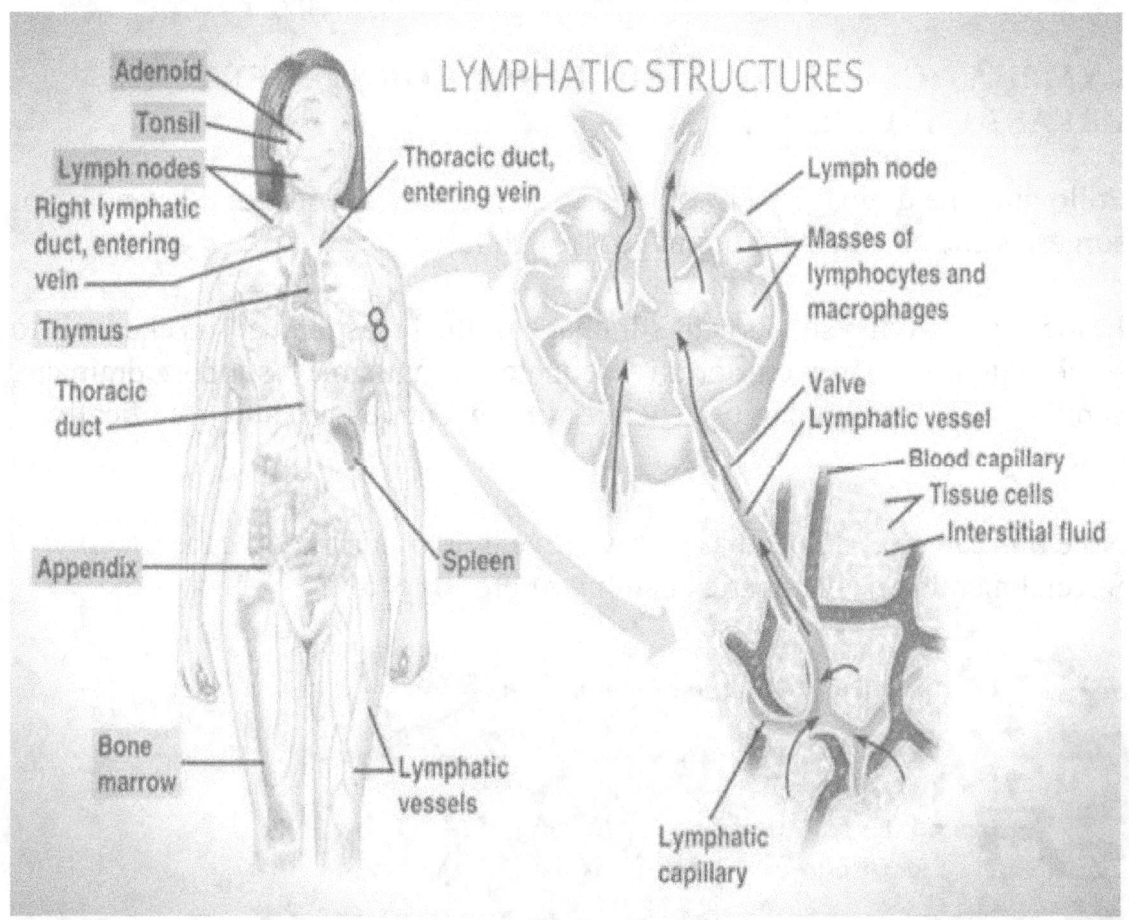

LASER LYMPHATIC DRAINAGE MAY BE VERY EFFECTIVE AT THE INITIAL STAGES

Plan a treatment based on

Age

Gender

Area

Stage

Position

Supporting therapies and drugs

Laser apparatus available
Repair of capillaries and nodes
Quantity in litres to be drained per session

LYMPHATICS ARE THE MAIN TARGET OF SURGERY IN BREAST CANCER.

Following the drainage pathway and structure may support understanding of surgeries and channels for drainage through laser.

Emptying the axilla supports the drainage of the breast and all its channels to some extent. A laser cluster of adequate strength may support drainage, capillary tone and immunity generally in preventive care and specifically in case of disease.

Note this can be developed as a preventive therapy for breast cancer
Special mention of lymphatic anatomy of breast region

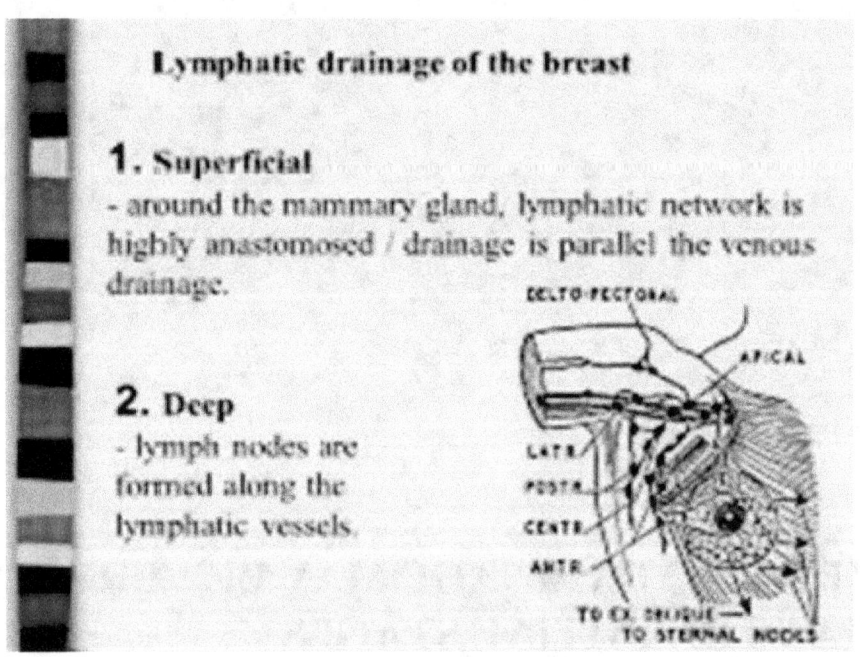

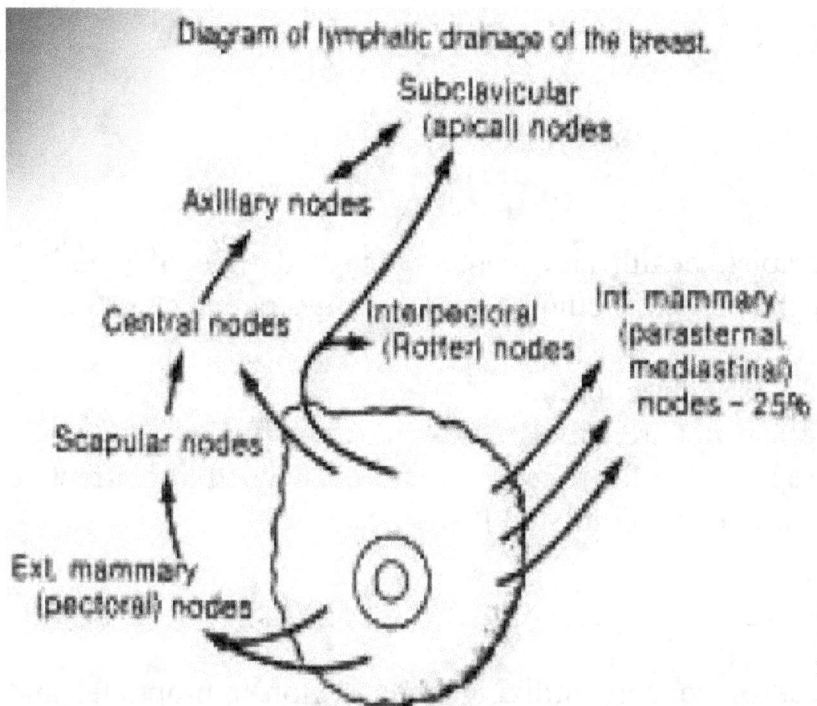

Diagram of lymphatic drainage of the breast.

The direction of lymph needed with laser must be assessed to determine the precise node to be fed.

This can be developed and assessed in the SOAP

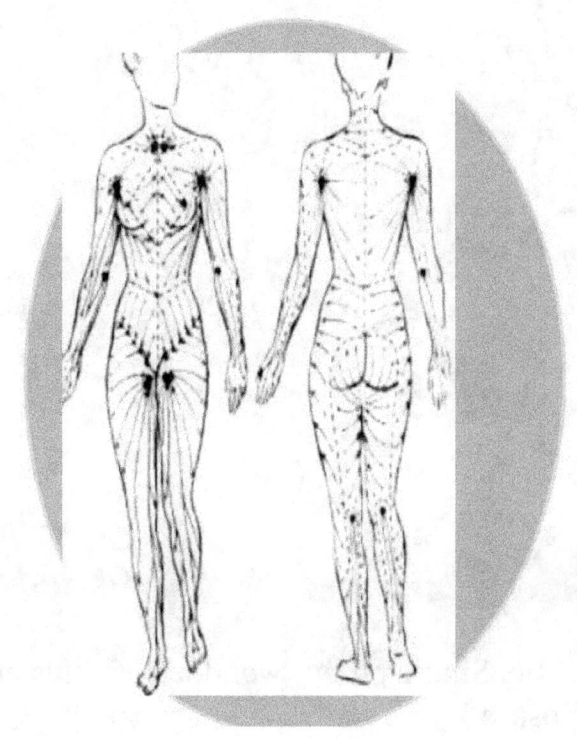

4.14. SOAP FOR LYMPHATICS

S   Daily SOAP Notes

LYMPHATICS
Name of patient, therapist, health care center, date and time of meeting. Details as reported by the patient should be marked in a separate chart

O   Draw arrows for Lymph direction
Mark the nodes to be flushed. Circle the areas with excess lymph
Manage to indicate repetition of strokes or duration needed for effective drainage based on quantity of accumulated fluid.

A __Therapists name_____, Laser lymphatic drainage
treated the above areas of concern utilizing body region appropriate, and patient
condition/tolerance appropriate, massage strokes and techniques. The laser/manual therapy was preformed from _____ am/pm to _____ am/pm on the above captioned date.

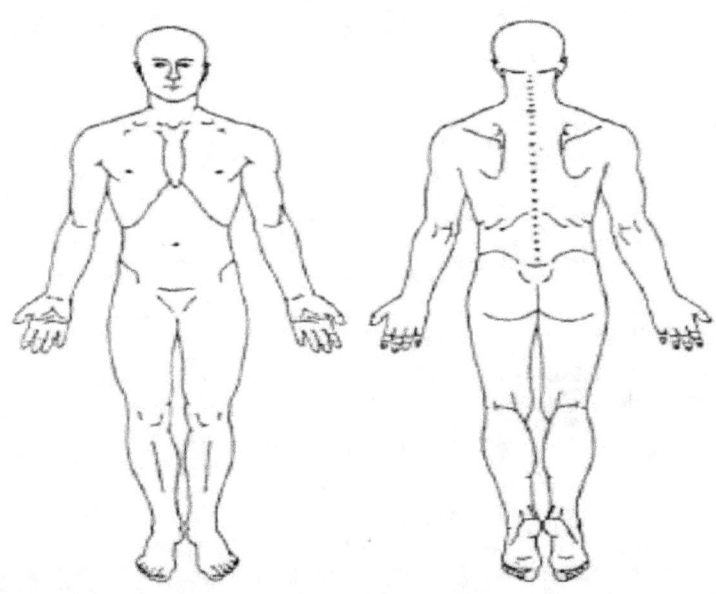

P   – Laser Therapy Techniques (ie. Single probe -woodpecker, cluster probe- scanning or stationary exposure).

Duration of exposure and dosage per area. Adjunct therapies – manual, hydrotherapy, heat, body wrap, other.

Patient/Client is to return: ☐ as needed ☐ per doctor's orders for follow up
_____

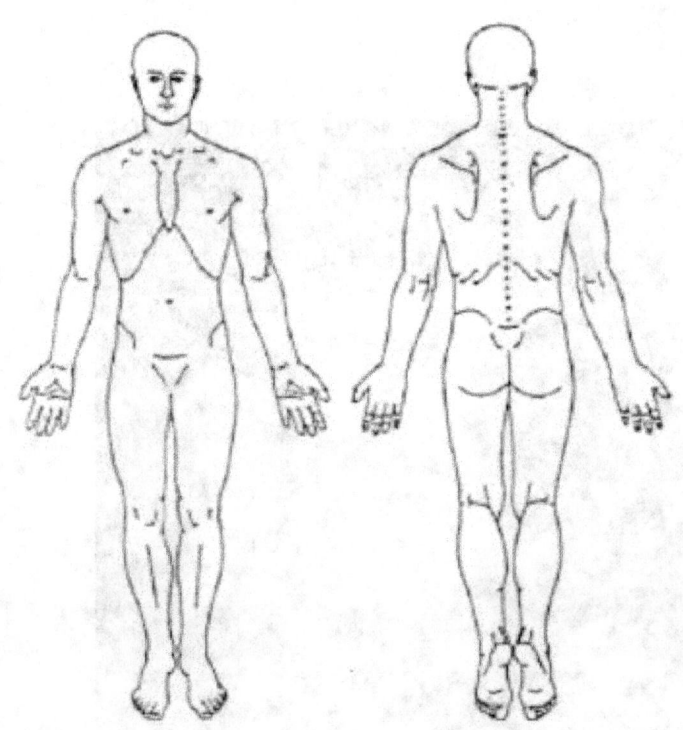

SECTION FIVE

LASER ACUPUNCTURE
THE NATURE OF ACUPUNCTURE POINTS
POINT SELECTION PROTOCOLS

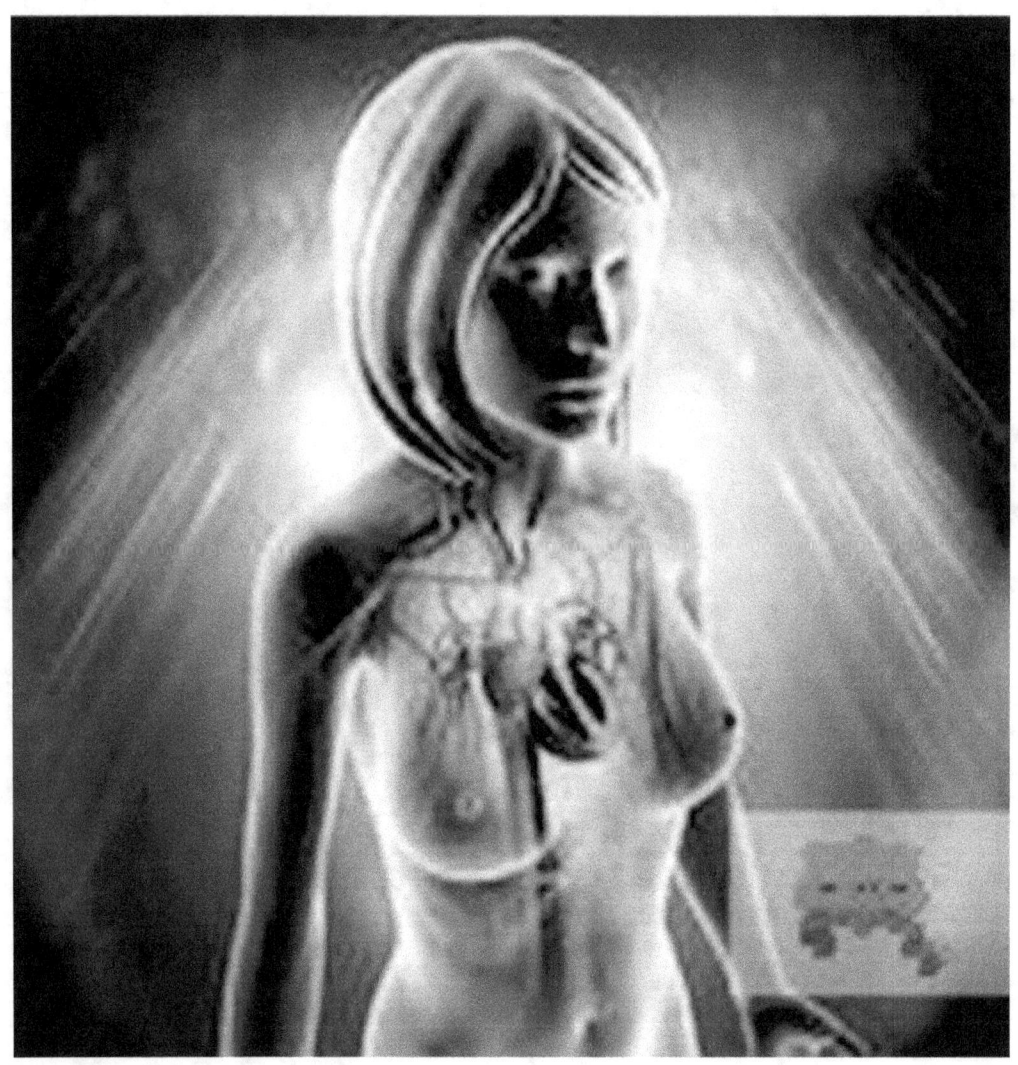

MICROACUPUNCTURE
LASER ACUPUNCTURE FREQUENCIES

SKILLS DEVELOPMENT IN THIS SECTION

KNOWLEDGE OF ACUPUNCTURE POINTS USED COMMONLY
WITH LASER
PRINCIPLES OF APPLICATION
MICROACUPUNCTURE TECHNIQUES
SELECTION OF LASER FREQUENCIES FOR POINTS
WALT DOSE RECOMMENDATIONS

CONTENTS

5.1 THE NATURE OF ACUPUNCTURE POINTS

Acupuncture point stimulation triggers a response in the CNS (opposed to TR pts which belong to the PNS).

Acupuncture points, upon stimulation, have shown a stronger pattern of firing in the hypothalamus than stimulation of non-acupuncture areas.

Acupuncture points in one of the many theories, are considered to be foci of embryonic origin, around which other cells and body parts developed. They therefore influence the meridian and the body area more comprehensively than non-acupuncture treatments. They have micro representation in miniature as in the hands, feet and ear. They also have pervasive and systemic influence.

Dr Nogier of France developed research on the embryonic origin of the points and frequencies in laser reactive to embryonic endodermal, mesodermal or ectodermal tissue.

Acupuncture science is several thousand years old, and belongs to China as a legacy from an evolved saint. The texts are complex to interpret. Modern science in laser acupuncture is based on rational scientific enquiry, and knowledge outcomes that are understood by practitioners to support medical therapies.

Apart from points and their descriptions, Classical acupuncture theory is based on meridians and five elements which will not be discussed much in this course.

Approaches to five element theory and diagnostics for treatment requires a multiple probe laser for applying to the YIN and Yang point simultaneously to achieve meridian balance. Excess is drained and deficiency is reinforced. This treatment requires classical assessment of symptoms and personality which are non-medical for our purpose. Although we have every respect for practitioners of this system.

Acupuncture points in thermography, show up as 'hot spots, with low electrical resistance in comparison to the surrounding sites.

Some authors have found that AP's coincide with TP's. Others have found differences in the nature of both. Both TP's and AP's are significant in therapy.

5.2 POINT SELECTION PROTOCOLS

1. AH SHI POINTS

These are points in close proximity to an injured area or pathological organ that develop tenderness so that the patient expresses pain AH when pressure is applied. These points are different from TP's as they belong to the CNS. They are highly reactive and curative in treatments and must be listed in treatment protocols.

5.3. BACK SHU POINTS

These are para vertebral points belonging to the Bladder meridian which lies 3 cms lateral to the dorsal midline between T3 and S4. They are reflex (SHU) points for the organs as under.

- T3 - T7: Lung. Pericardium, Heart, Governor Vessel (and spine), Diaphragm (and blood).

- T9 - T12: Liver, Gallbladder, Spleen (and blood/immunity), Stomach.

- L1 – L5: Triple Heater (Endocrine/respiration/digestion/elimination), Kidney, Large Intestine

-S1 – S4: Small Intestine, Bladder

In disorders of the organs or limbs, the relevant Shu point of the corresponding dermatome becomes sensitive.

Tender Shu points are given along with AH SHI points and TP points for therapies involving management of pain, and increased range of motion.

5.4 FRONT MU POINTS

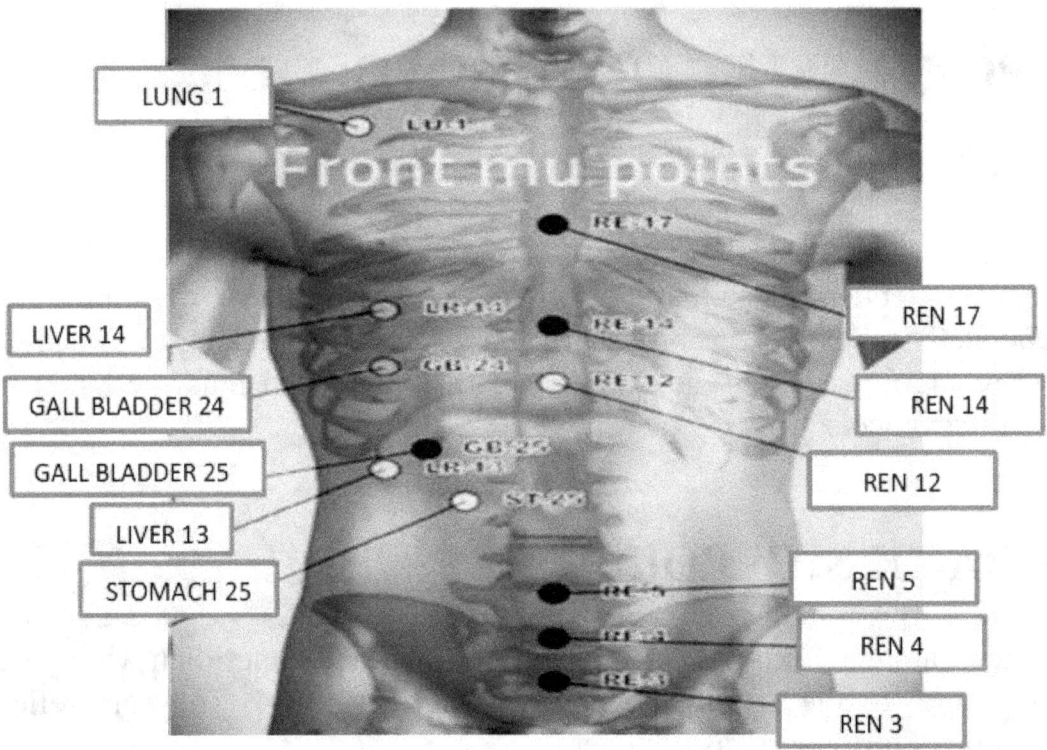

These are points belonging to the central line in the front side, reflecting organ pathologies

A front Mu Yin point has a corresponding Back Shu Yang point. These point combinations are sometimes chosen to sort out organ disorders as Asthma, or liver diseases.

LIVER 14
GALL BLADDER 24
GALL BLADDER 25
LIVER 13
STOMACH 25
LUNG 1
REN 17
REN 14
REN 12

REN 5
REN 4
REN 3

Pressure applied to tender points may be extremely painful in its reflex action and yet give fast relief. These points radiate deep into the pathological organ.

5.5 MICROACUPUNCTURE

The body has full body representation in hands, feet and the ear. These techniques are known under Auricular therapy, and Korean Hand Therapy (KHT.)

Yamamoto scalp acupuncture also uses laser on some of the points that are therapeutic in the microsystem. These techniques are specialized and only some will be discussed in this course that have maximum relevance to laser therapy

5.6 MORE ON SHU - SEGMENTAL PARAVERTEBRAL POINTS

In myofascial pain, paravertebral Ah SHI points may be found alongside TPs in tender muscles.

These paravertebral points correlate with SHU points in TCM. In autonomic dysfunctions these back SHU points have often a segmental connection to corresponding inner organs. These segmental AH SHI points and SHU points will give maximum relief to musculoskeletal disorders when the disease lies in more than just a taut muscle band. Treatment may be combined with local treatment protocols for maximum effectiveness.

Ah Shi points are of two kinds
- Those that refer pain

- Those that do not refer pain.

Physical therapists may check to see the nature of the Ah Shi point and decide on the likely outcome of laser treatment.

Physical therapists must also recheck after treatment to assess through palpation or electrical resistance point detector, the changes that have taken place.

These points are only effective in therapy if they are tender.

5.7 EXACT LOCATION OF POINTS

Points may be located by

1. Applying pressure
Pressure tolerance is important for assessment, for selection of points,
and a tool to determine progress. Scales from 1 – 10 may be recorded, even before and after treatment.
Fit athletes have better a higher pain threshold than unfit persons.
Men have a higher pain threshold than women.
Functional disorders have lower pressure tolerance than organic disease.
2. Use of electrical resistance meter
3. These are probes that sometimes accompany lasers, with a resistance meter that detects points of low electrical resistance. The probe is applied at right angles to the skin at continuous pressure and moved over suspected area.

These resistance meters are also called point finders, and may be used for the body or auricle.

Points known to respond to laser acupuncture - recommended by Prof Pontinen.

Code Location

GV 20	Vertex
BL 57	Calf
TE 21	Face
GB 20	Neck

LI 4 Hand

SI 3 Hand
GB 30 Buttock
ST 6 Face
GB 21 Shoulder
TE 14 Shoulder
LI 15 Shoulder
ST 41 Ankle joint
BL 60 Ankle
PC 6 Arm
CV 6 Abdomen
LI 11 Arm
SP 6 Leg
BL 23 Back
LI 10 Arm
LR 3 Foot
Ex HN 5 Face
ST 38 Leg
TE 15 Shoulder
TE 5 arm
BL 54 Fossa polpitea
ST 7 Face
BL 15 Back
Ex LE 5 Knee
GB 34 Leg
LI 5 Hand
Sp 9 leg
CV 12 abdomen
St 36 leg

All back Shu points and front mu points must be managed for deep treatment and best results. Whereas either mu or Shu point provides therapeutic relief if tender or indicated, both points combined improve recovery downtime.

Back Shu and front mu points are listed below:

Front Mu Points Chart

Lung	LU 1	Urinary Bladder	CV 3
Large Intestine	ST 25	Kidney	GB 25
Stomach	CV 12	Pericardium	CV 17
Spleen	LV 13	Triple Heater	CV 5
Heart	CV 14	Gall Bladder	GB 24
Small Intestine	CV 4	Liver	LV 14

Back Shu Points Theory and Applications

Used primarily to treat their related organ, especially with chronic conditions.

May be used for problems in the local area.

Used diagnostically as they often become sore when their related organ is imbalanced.

Some historical texts point more to their usage as treating imbalances within the yin organs, while the Front Mu points will treat imbalances within the yang organs.

Back Shu Points Chart

Lung	UB 13	Urinary Bladder	UB 28
Large Intestine	UB 25	Kidney	UB 23
Stomach	UB 21	Pericardium	UB 14
Spleen	UB 20	Triple Heater	UB 22
Heart	UB 15	Gall Bladder	UB 19
Small Intestine	UB 27	Liver	UB 18
Governing Vessel	UB 16	Diaphragm	UB 17
Qihai (Sea of Qi)	UB 24	Guanyuan (Gate of Source)	UB 26
Zhonglu (Center Back Muscles)	UB 29	Baihuan (White Ring)	UB 30
Gaohuang (Vital Region)	UB 43		

COMMAND POINTS

There are certain command points that influence energetic of the region they command.

These points may improve the effects of laser therapy in the area if they are stimulated as a part of treatment protocols. They are used frequently and given importance as points that treat any disorders belonging to this region

These are

LI 4 : Influence mouth and face
LU 7 : Neck and head
ST 36: Abdomen
BL 40 : Back
P 6 : Chest
Du 26 : Mind

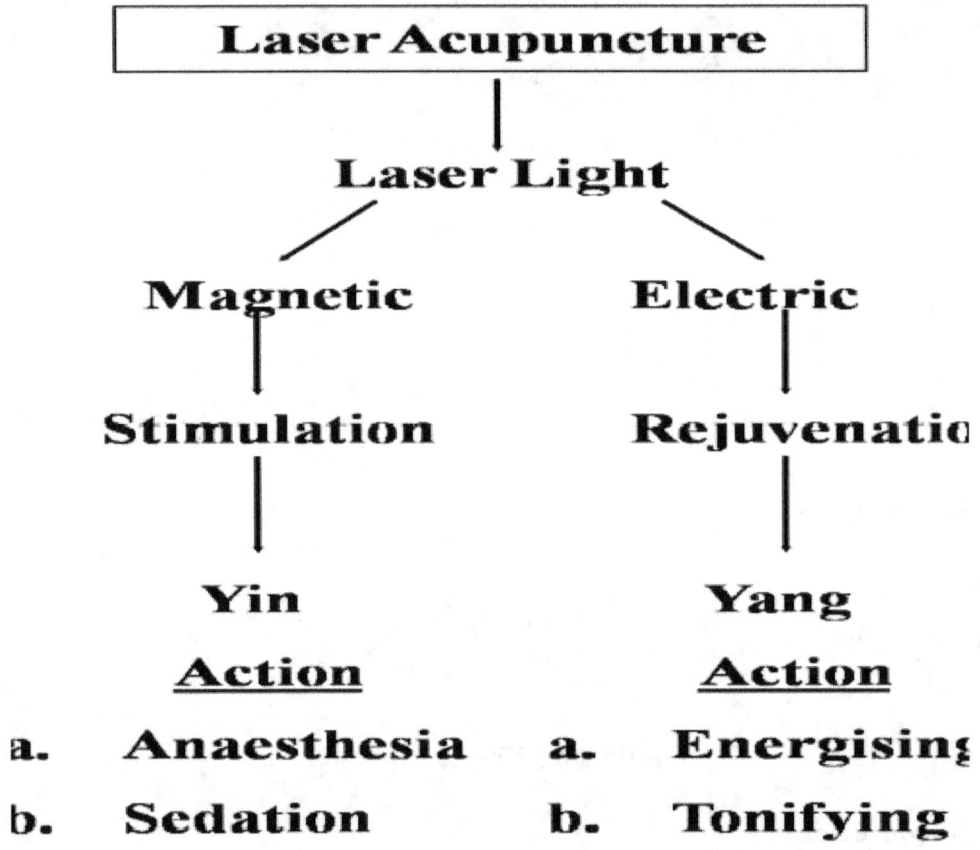

In addition GV 20 and Kidney 1 are used in combination for calming effects and for providing latent energy for the body to heal itself with all treatments. These points may be used in emergency, or when there are multiple complications.

The chart above shows Yin protocols for sedation and analgesia. This involves large dose of laser. Energizing and tonifying doses are shorter and are yang in nature.

The same points and point combinations must be prepared according to the sedation or tonification requirement of the treatment.

Incase the therapist is not well acquainted with acupuncture energetics, they can still rely on palpation for tenderness and pain, and on client observation, before and after the treatment.

POINT COMBINATIONS OF INTEREST

SP 4 is combined with P 6 to treat diseases of the heart, stomach or chest.

LU 7 is combined with K 6 to treat diseases of the lung, chest, diaphragm or throat.

SJ 5 is combined with GB 41 to treat diseases of the ear, neck, shoulder or cheek.

SI 3 is combined with Bl 62 to treat diseases of the inner can thus, neck or shoulder.

Liv 3 is combined with LI 4 to reduce pain anywhere in the body.

GV 20 is combined with K 1 for deep effects and therapeutic potentials.

These are only some important point combinations.

5.6 MICROACUPUNCTURE

The auricle, hands and feet have been known in ancient science, to represent the human body in miniature. These are projection zones which have been investigated in great details by pioneers as Dr Nogier of France, and Dr Bahr of Germany. These schools of thought developed laser frequencies specific to embryonic tissue, and to related zones of the body.

Lasers frequently have Nogier frequencies. These have been listed in section 1. Some more details are below.

Sedatelec lasers has presented that seven electro frequencies were developed experimentally by Dr Paul Nogier in the 1970s. These frequencies are constantly used in routine medical practice, as they are preferentially recognized by the body. They enter into resonance with some biological receptors and specific exert effects on the body. These frequencies are used both for detection and for treatment.

Frequencies U A B C D E F G
Value (Hz) 1.14 2.28 4.56 9.125 18.25 36.5 73 146
The U frequency is the so-called "universal" frequency and the resulting 7 fundamental frequencies are multiples of 2.

Later the same frequencies became important for laser devices, but at a higher harmonic. They have an identical action. These have since been widely used by laser manufacturers, especially for equine treatments.

However the frequencies are valid only in relation to

Acupuncture. They were based on research that showed normalization of the pulse when acupuncture was given with the specific frequency

Frequencies A B C D E F G
Value (Hz) 292 584 1168 2336 4672 73 146

Variations with respect to reference frequencies are also used. They range from -30% to +30%.

Embryonic categories have become diagnostic and evaluative measures for energy therapists to consult with clients. There are ectodermal, endodermal and mesodermal types of physique and client types. However we are interested only in identifying with the relation of the embryonic tissue to the laser frequency and the point selection. The rules are general and the Learner must struggle to improve skills in this field.

The works of Nogier has greatly influenced developments in medical acupuncture. The ability to manage embryonic tissue provides a new dimension to therapy as embryonic tissues form connective fascial links to the entire body. The capacity for micro treatments and distant therapy triggers emerges from the discovery of this active fascial web that influences every aspect of the physique and its response to treatment. Apart from embryonic tissue controls through the micro acupuncture points, it has also been discovered that the vagus nerve of the ear releases powerful hormones as leptin, which influences body mass, weight and metabolism.

Definition of frequencies by Drs Paul and Raphaël Nogier:
Extract from "The man in the ear", Maisonneuve, 1979, 255 p.

The "A" frequency is associated, in the animal kingdom, with non-organized, embryonic structures. It is the frequency of the primitive living being; it is in sympathy with the cell in the crude, undifferentiated state. This frequency, the most archaic, can also be considered to be the most anarchic.

The more elaborate "B" frequency is specific to the nutritional visceral system and is related to the primitive gastrointestinal apparatus.
The "C" frequency indicates motor elements of the body. It reflects movement, the limbs, the renal system, the genital tract.

The "D" frequency leads us to a higher level of organization, as it introduces the concept of symmetry, by selectively affecting certain unpaired organs, presenting the characteristic of being solitary, but anatomically symmetrical; for example the corpus callosum or the white commissure, two symmetrical cerebral structures, situated between the right hemisphere and the left hemisphere [...]

The "E" frequency is that of the spinal cord and central nervous system, which perceives and communicates between functional units situated at different levels.

The "F" frequency represents subcortical cerebral regions. These structures are found in the brain of higher animals, dogs, for example.

The "G" frequency resonates with the most elaborate structures of the body, those of the cerebral cortex, the typically human part of the brain, which gives man the capacity to think, create and imagine.

The following table summarizes the main therapeutic applications of Nogier frequencies:

Freq. **THERAPEUTIC POTENTIAL**

A Action on the tissues wounds, epithelial tumours, epidermal reactions...

B Gastrointestinal and metabolic problems trophic functions, polarity, parasympathetic, impulses...

C Loco motor problems ergo tropic function, sympathetic polarity....

D Disorders of laterality

E Pain and nerve conduction spinal cord diseases

F Brain and bone reconstruction

G Action on the cerebral cortex cortical, mental disorders...

The effects can be potentiated by associating various frequencies. These combinations of frequencies are especially used in local therapy:

TREATMENT ANALGESIC REGENERATING MUSCLE RELAXING
Frequencies E G A B F C D G

NOGIER FREQUENCIES INVOLVE
-Frequency
-Disease
-Part of the Body
-Point

A'/292
Acute illness, cellular level, inflammation, tumours
Body orifices. Shu point

B'/584
Chronic illness, metabolism, cell nutrition
Abdomen
Sedation

C'/1168
Circulation, energy transfer, loco motor disorders
Bones, muscles, joints, extremities tonification

D'/2336
Psychic disorders, fatigue, laterality disorders
Commissures
Alarm point

E'/4672
Nerve disturbances/pain, neuralgia, neuritides
Spinal cord, nerves
Starting point
F'/9344
Depressions, psychic symptoms and causes, bone reconstruction
Face, sub cortex, emotions. End point

G'/18688
Intellectual and psychosomatic disturbances
Frontal cerebral zone
Source point

The shaded charts below indicate auricular frequency correlations in the

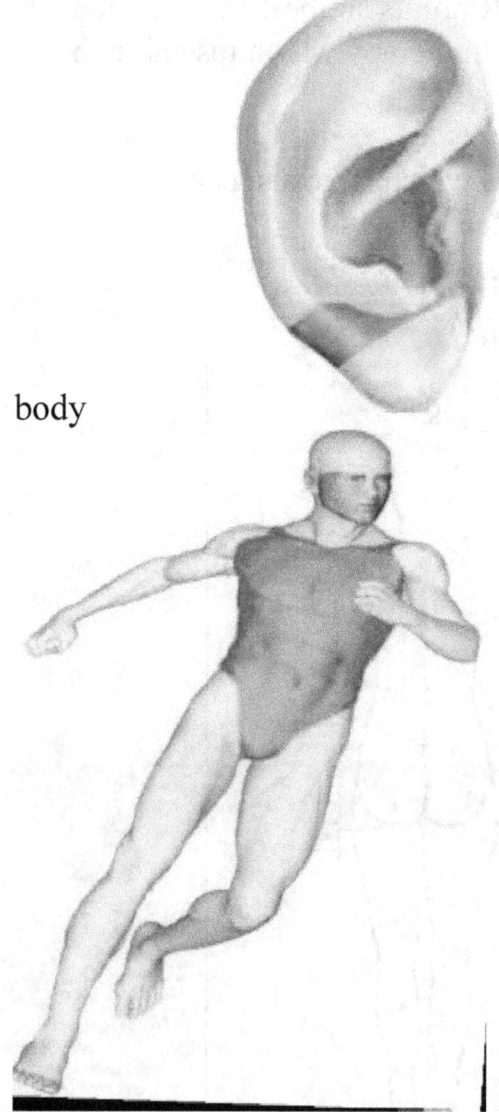

body

From Sedatelec, a laser manufacturing company in France belonging to Dr Nogiers methodology

A = Orange
B = Red
C = yellow
D = dark pink
E = Blue
F = Light pink

G = purple

According to Nogier, the auricular MASTER points are best treated with laser. These points have a general influence in therapy which resemble their name.

Alongside are also organ, or structural points which have a specific influence on therapy. Images are from Sedatelec lasers.

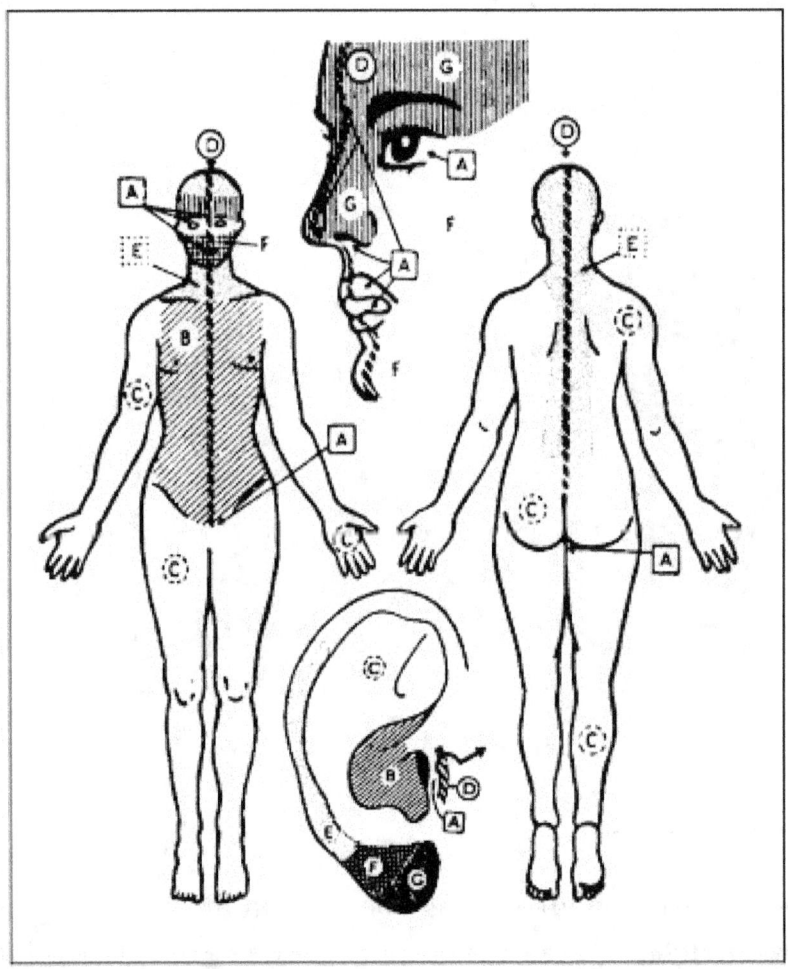

Charts provided indicate 15 master points and 15 specific points. Nogier points are generally separate from Chinese points as they are based on scientific understanding whereas Chinese points are mythological. Nogier points combine well with body treatments. 10 important master auricular points are discussed below.

Point Zero

Homeostatic Balance; Returns body to the idealized state which was present in the womb; Autonomic Brain that controls visceral organs via peripheral nerve ganglia; Supports other auricular points

Shen Men
Tranquilizes the Mind - allows connection to spirit; Alleviates stress, pain, tension, anxiety, depression, insomnia, restlessness, excessive sensitivity; Reduces cough, fever, inflammation, blood pressure, epilepsy; Supports other auricular points.

Autonomic Point
(Sympathetic)
Balances the activity of the sympathetic and parasympathetic nervous systems; vasodilator to improve blood circulation; Relieves stress-related health disorders

Thalamus Point
Control Point)
Restores tranquillity by regulating over-excitement and restraining the cerebral cortex; Reduces Pain

Endocrine Point
(Pituitary Gland)
Homeostasis of Hormone; Anti-inflammatory, alleviates hypersensitivity, rheumatism, and urogenital disorders
Master
Oscillation
Point
Balances the left and right hemispheres to treat dyslexia, learning disability, ADD

Allergy Point
Reduces inflammation related to allergy, rheumatoid arthritis, asthma; Stimulates removal of toxic substances and metabolic waste; Anaphylactic shock.

Tranquilizer Point

Sedative; Relaxation; Alleviates general anxiety; Reduces
High blood pressure, Chronic stress

Master Sensorial
(Eye Point)
Controls sensory cerebral cortex of parietal, temporal, occipital; Reduces unpleasant/excessive sensation (tactile paraesthesia, tinnitus, blurred vision, diabetic neuropathy)

Master Cerebral
(Neurasthenia)
Represents the pre-frontal lobe, which makes decisions & initiates conscious action. Alleviates anxiety, fever, worry; Alleviates OCD, Psychosomatic disorders; Relieves Negative-Pessimistic Thinking that accompanies chronic pain.

Master Points on the Ear by Professor Hanah Koh

A. **Point Zero** (Midear)
This master point is the geometrical and physiological centre of the whole auricle. It brings the whole body towards homeostasis, producing a balance of energy, hormones, and brain activity. It supports the actions of other auricular points and returns the body to the idealized state which was present in the womb. On the auricular soma topic map, Point Zero is located where the umbilical cord would rise from the abdomen of the inverted foetus pattern found on the ear. As the solar plexus point, Point Zero serves as the autonomic brain that controls visceral organs through peripheral nerve ganglia.

B. **Shenmen** (Neurogate)
The purpose of Shenmen is to tranquilize the mind and to allow harmonious connection essential spirit. This master point alleviates stress, pain, tension, anxiety, depression, insomnia, restlessness, and excessive sensitivity. The Chinese believe that Shenmen affects excitation and inhibition of the cerebral cortex, and excessive sensitivity. Nogier's 2nd phase Thalamus point is localized to the same area of the ear. It is utilized in almost all treatment plans, including acupuncture analgesia for surgery.

Shemen was one of the 1st points emphasized for the detoxification from drugs and the treatment of alcoholism and substance abuse. It is also used to reduce coughs, fever, inflammatory disease, epilepsy, and high blood pressure. When it is difficult to find tender or electrically active ear points, stimulation of either Shenmen or Point Zero increases the reactivity of other auricular points, making it easier to detect them.

C. Sympathetic Autonomic Point

This master point balances the sympathetic nervous system activation with parasympathetic sedation. This point is the primary ear locus for diagnosing visceral pain and for inducing sedation effects during acupuncture. It improves blood circulation by facilitating vasodilation, corrects irregular or rapid heartbeats, reduces angina pain, alleviates Raymond's diseases, reduces visceral pain from internal organs, calms smooth muscle spasms, and reduces neurovegetativ disequilibrium. It is also used for the treatment of KD stones, gallstones, gastric ulcers, abdominal distention, asthma, and dysfunctions of the autonomic nervous system.

D. Allergy Point

This master point leads to a general reduction in inflammatory reactions related to allergies, rheumatoid arthritis, and asthma. It is used for the elimination of toxic substances, the excretion of metabolic wastes, and treatment of anaphylactic shock. In oriental medicine, the top surface of the allergy point is pricked with a needle to reduce excess qi, or it is pinched to diminish allergic reactions.

E. Thalamus Point (Subcortex, Brain, Pain Control Point)

This master point represents the whole diencephalons, including the thalamus and the hypothalamus. It affects thalamic relay connections to the cerebral cortex and hypothalamic regulation of autonomic nerves and endocrine glands. The thalamus is the highest level of the supraspinal gate control system, and so is used for most pain disorders, acute and chronic, and is frequently used for auricular acupuncture analgesia. It also reduces neurasthenia, anxiety, depression, schizophrenia, overexcitement, sweating, swelling, shock, nausea, gastritis, hypertension, coronary disorders, vomiting, diarrhea, constipation, LV disorders, and GB dysfunctions.

In TCM, the Thalamus Subcortex Point tonifies the brain and calms the mind. In the Nogier phase system, the Phase II Thalamus is located in the region of Shenmen, and Phase III

Thalamus is located in the region of the LU. These 3 points, Thalamus, Shenmen, and LU, are all used for drug detoxification.

F. **Endocrine Point** (Internal Secretion Pituitary Gland)
This master point brings endocrine hormones to their appropriate homeostatic levels, either raising or lowering glandular secretions. It functions by activating the pituitary gland below the brain. The pituitary is the master gland controlling all other endocrine glands. It relives hypersensitivity, rheumatism, hyperthyroidism, diabetes mellitus, irregular menstruation, sexual dysfunction, and urogenital disorders. It has anti-allergic, anti-rheumatic, and anti-inflammatory effects. In TCM treatments, it reduces dampness and relieves swelling and oedema.

G. **Oscillation Point** (Laterality Point, Switching Point)
This master point balances laterality disorders related to the left and right cerebral hemispheres. Anatomically it represents the corpus callosum and the anterior commissure.

The point is active in the people who are left-handed or mixed dominant in handedness.

Whereas 80% of individuals show ipsilateral representation of body organs, 20% exhibit contralateral representation. These individuals are viewed as oscillators in the European School of Auriculotherapy, and this laterality dysfunction is labelled "switched" in somechiropractic schools. Stimulation of this auricular point in oscillators is often necessary before any other active auriculotherapy treatment on the contralateral ear may become more conducive on the ipsilateral ear. This point is used to alleviate dyslexia, learning disabilities, and ADD. People who have unusual or hypersensitive reactions to prescription medications or auto immune problems often need to be treated for oscillation.

H. **Tranquilizer Point** (Valium Analog Point, Hypertensive Point)
This master point produces a general sedation effect, facilitating overall relaxation and relieving generalized anxiety. It also reduces high blood pressure and chronic stress.

I. **Sensorial Point** (Eye Point)

This point controls the sensory cerebral cortex area of the parietal, temporal, and occipital lobes. It is used to reduce any unpleasant or excessive sensation, such as parasthesia, tinnitus, and blurred vision.

J. Cerebral Point (Master Omega, Nervousness, Neurasthenia, Worry). This master point represents the prefrontal lobe of the brain, the part of the cerebral cortex which makes decisions and initiates conscious action. Stimulation of this auricular point diminishes nervous anxiety, fever, worry, lassitude, dream-disturbed sleep, poor memory, obsessive-compulsive disorders, psychosomatic disorders, and negative pessimistic thinking which often accompanies chronic pain problems.

K. **Adrenal Point**
This master point releases the hormone adrenaline in response to activation bysympathetic nerves and adrenal cortex, which release cortisol and other stress related hormone in response to pituitary adrenocorticotropic hormone (ACTH).

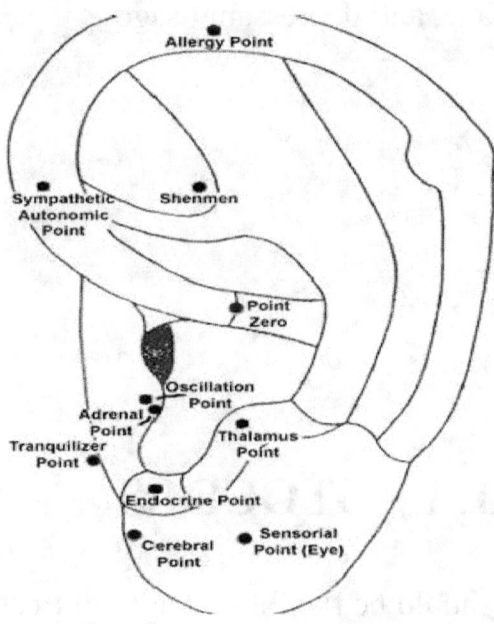

Representation in the Ear in its somatotopy is logical

-In the center is the concha, which is innervated by the vagus nerve, contains the point locations of the tissues derived from the ENDODERM

-In the middle region, the antihelix and a part of the helix is innervated by the trigeminal nerve, corresponding to points derived from tissues of the MESODERM

-In the peripheral area, a part of the helix and the lobe innervated by the superficial cervical plexus contain the point locations of tissues of the ECTODERM.

INDICATIONS FOR AURICULOTHEAPY

Pain
Metabolic, traumatic, neurological
Functional disorders:
:Tachycardia, constipation, irritable bowel syndrome, chronic fatigue

Disorders of dependency
: Tobacco addiction, tranquilizer usage, anti depressant usage

Psychological disorder
: Reactive depression Anxiety

Dermatological disorder
: Eczema, Psoriasis, Alopecia

Contraindications
: Pregnancy

5.7 LASER PUNCTURE PROTOCOLS

Laser puncture treatment protocols should be flexible. Length of treatment will vary with the wavelength and power output of the laser and the body part being treated. Variations of Nogier's frequencies are commonly used for laser-puncture . In general, the lower the wavelength of the laser, the longer the treatment time at each point.
All commonly used types of therapeutic lasers can be used for laser puncture (GaAlAs, and GAAs diodes; see Figures 10-12). The usual treatment times

range between 15–20 seconds for an infrared GAAs or GaAlAs laser. Higher power outputs of the laser will shorten treatment times on each point. A low output laser (5–20mW) may require 30–60 seconds per point. A medium output laser (50–250mW) may require 10–20 seconds per point. A high output laser (500mW or more) may require only 5–10 seconds per point.

Total treatment times for all the points treated at that session would be somewhere between 2 and 4 minutes.

Professor Pontinen has found in his scientific investigations that acupuncture points of high sensitivity and low electrical resistance must be treated with radiation of a reduced dose to about 0.1- 0.2 J/pt., i.e. 10% of the normal dose of treatment of muscle Trigger points which respond to 1 – 2 J/pt.
An inhibitory dose (longer exposure) has to be given on acute and painful conditions, and a stimulatory dose(short exposure) in chronic conditions with deficiencies as to improve immunity, improve tissue strength, proliferate fibroblasts.

Standard dosage levels

G. Danhof

Analgesic effect in the treatment of muscular pain

Dosage	2-4 joules/cm²
Therapy time	40-80 seconds

Analgesic effect in the treatment of painful joints

Dosage	4-8 joules/cm²
Therapy time	80-160 seconds

Acute inflammation

Dosage	1-6 joules/cm²
Therapy time	20-120 seconds

Chronic inflammation

Dosage	4-8 joules/cm¹
Therapy time	80-160 seconds

Stimulation of the metabolism

Dosage	3-6 joules/cm²
Therapy time	80-120 seconds

Stimulation of blood circulation

Dosage	1-3 joules/cm²
Therapy time	20-60 seconds

All
values are rough guidelines and should be adapted to suit the individual
case. Further information can be found in:

Clinical Laser Therapy, by J.Kert & L.Rose,
Lasertherapie bijSportblessures, by G. Danhof

Koel, Moolenaar, en Castel

Dermatology

Scars (too soft)	3-6 J/cm²
Scars (painful keloids)	0,5-1 J/cm²
Decubitus	0,1-2 J/cm²
Ulcus	0,1-2 J/cm²
Transplantation wounds	0,1-1J/cm²

Rheumatic/orthopaedic

Tendinitis/peritendinitis	0,5-4 J/cm²
Periostalgia	0,5-2 J/cm²
Bursitis	0,5-2 J/cm²
Fasciatis plantaris	0,3-1 J/cm²
Capsulitis	0,5-3 J/cm²
Myositis	0,5-2 J/cm²

Posttraumatic treatment

Distortions	0,5-2 J/cm²
Rupture	0,5-3 J/cm²
Haematoma	0,5-3 J/cm²
Oedema	0,5-2 J/cm²

Neurology

Neuralgia	0,05-0,8 J/cm²
Neuritis	0,05-0,8 J/cm²

Taken from: Laser Therapy for Sports Injuries.

RJ does not recommend such low energy levels. We think that the energy should be at least between 2-5 Joule on pale skin and higher dosage on dark skin.

5.8 EXPERTS ON ACUPUNCTURE

In fact, Enwemeka has stated on LIGHT. The present view is that light has a dual character. In its propagation it consists of electromagnetic waves, but when it interacts with matter in emission, absorption and scattering processes we must consider it as composed of photons. The photo-acupuncture process consists of the emission of light from a semiconductor chip, its scattering through the flesh and absorption into the nervous system, so it can only be sensibly described as a stream of photons. Terms such as coherence and collimation describe waves, not particles, so are meaningless with photons.

When a photon decays, it becomes an electron with the same energy level. In photo-puncture, most photons decay in the tissues, but those which encounter the acupuncture point stimulate it electrically, thus sending patterns of stimuli to the brain. Photons are fundamental particles and differ from each

The present view other only in their energy level, i.e. their perceived colour. A red photon from a laser is identical with a red photon from a Gallium Aluminium Arsenide chip or from a burning match. Ascribing other properties to them would probably be contrary to modern physics. The objective is to achieve levels of stimulation which the brain cannot ignore.
With the previous technology, the only practical way of generating intense red or infrared light strong enough for the brain to recognize was a gas (helium-neon) laser or a solid state laser. In order to get a useful power output, it was necessary to pass high current pulses through these
devices. With the latest technology, this is no longer necessary for high light output.

The nervous system works by an interchange of sodium $Na+$ and potassium $K+$ ions, a slow process which could never follow these high pulse rates. What has been demonstrated is that the end effect depends upon the total energy into the acupuncture point. This can be mechanical. Heat, electrical, chemical. Sound, magnetic or here, light energy. It has to be above
a certain threshold, or the brain ignores it, so the rate at which the energy is injected by the time of application is the key to success.

5.9 SOAP FOR LAP

Care must be taken to be seen to be listening; full attention needs to be given to the person who is speaking. More detailed notes can be written whilst the patient is preparing for the treatment or between appointments. The consultation is an essential part of the healing process. Patients appreciate the time and attention being paid to their problem. The more patients understand and are involved the more comfortable they are likely to be with their treatment. Copies of the patients chart and treatment plan can easily be given or sent on to the patient if required. Treatment Record Systems A number of treatment record formats exist including SOAP and CARE notes.

The system you use doesn't need to be an acronym, you can adapt or develop your own format but it should satisfy certain minimum requirements.

Documentation is important as it –

Provides an examination and treatment history for each session.
Provides a record of contraindications and red flags.
Demonstrates and monitors patient progress.
Provides evidence to defend against a malpractice suit.
Provides records for reimbursement from insurance companies.
Provides records to be shared in the case of a referral.
It may be required by law or code of practice.

Client intake form
Name
D.O.B / Address/ Telephone/ Mobile/Email/Doctor's Address/Occupation/

Consent to examination and treatment. Template sample.

I understand the reasons for my examination and treatment and give my consent to these procedures being used by ....
(Therapist). I understand that records of my treatment will be kept in accordance with the Data Protection Act 1998 (UK) NS.O.A.P
Notes Subjective, objective, assessment and plan This is a common method of documentation used by health care professionals. It may be the advised method of documentation when dealing with insurance companies and will provide a familiar, consistent format when communicating with doctors and other health care workers.

SOAP

Subjective:
The patient's condition in their own words. Onset/History Location
Character of Pain (Sharp/Dull Ache)
Degree of Pain(1-10) Alleviating/Aggravating factors Temporal
pattern(Worse in the morning) Medical History(General health/Medication)
Social History(work/exercise) □

Objective:

Observation and testing Posture ROM Palpation Special Tests ☐
Assessment:
Evaluate the information
Summarize current status List relevant problems Post treatment assessment (changes) Patient response ☐ Plan: Address future treatments Exercises Special care instructions/ advice
Referral? Next appointment notes C.A.R.E Notes Condition of client, Action taken, Response of client, Evaluation Another system of documentation used by therapists. ☐ Condition of Client Subjective and objective assessment of client Current condition Areas of discomfort.
Medical/ Family History Emotional wellbeing Observations (posture/ degree of movement)
Palpation Degree of discomfort(1-10) ☐ Action taken: Summary of treatment and techniques used during session ☐ Response of Client: Feedback from client Verbal *response Nonverbal*
response ☐ Evaluation: An evaluation of the treatment and plans for future sessions
Overall assessment of session Advice/ suggestions given Follow up session notes/ treatment plan
Name................................. Signature..................................
Date........

S.O.A.P Notes

Subjective, objective, assessment and plan

Subjective:
The patient's condition in their own words.
Onset/History
Location
Character of Pain (Sharp/Dull Ache)
Degree of Pain(1-10)
Alleviating/Aggravating factors
Temporal pattern(Worse in the morning)
Medical History(General health/Medication)
Social History(work/exercise)

Objective:
Observation and testing
Posture

ROM
Palpation
Special Tests
Areas of body to be treated to manage frequency administration, and likely imbalance

Assessment:
Evaluate the information
Summarise current status
List relevant problems
Post treatment assessment (changes)
Patient response

Plan:
Markate any selection of auricular master points needed
Any selection of body points or influential points needed
If LAP is a combination laser treatment, or is being used by itself.
Decide on laser frequency needed
Decide on dosimetry
Decide on embryonic tissue correspondences.
Address future treatments
Exercises
Special care instructions/ advice
Referral?
Next appointment notes
C.A.R.E Notes
Condition of client, Action taken, Response of client, Evaluation
Another system of documentation used by therapists.
Condition of Client
Subjective and objective assessment of client
Current condition
Areas of discomfort
Medical/ Family History
Emotional wellbeing
Observations (posture/ degree of movement)
Palpation
Degree of discomfort(1-10)
 Action taken: Summary of treatment and techniques used during session
 Response of Client: Feedback from client
Verbal response

Nonverbal response
Evaluation: An evaluation of the treatment and plans for future sessions
Overall assessment of session
Advice/ suggestions given
Follow up session notes/ treatment plan

For **PLAN**
Chart out embryonic tissue correspondences, tender points in affected region, influential points, and laser frequencies, with dosimetry.

Rework this every session
Manage indicators on images

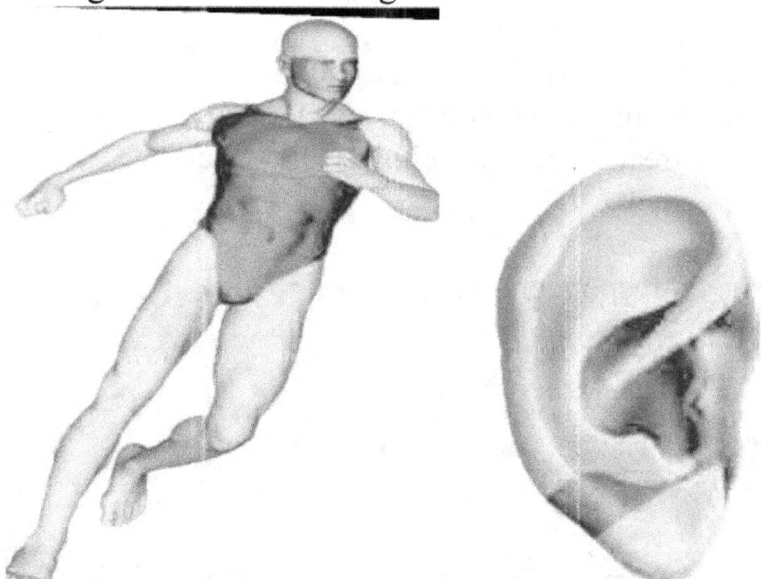

Laser Acupuncture evolution has migrated to the spectrums and sophisticated technologies of Weberneedles, that is used widely to manage several needle through fiber optic lasers at the time.

However scientific studies and commentaries are making a substantial impression on the arena, that endorses it for public practical usage.

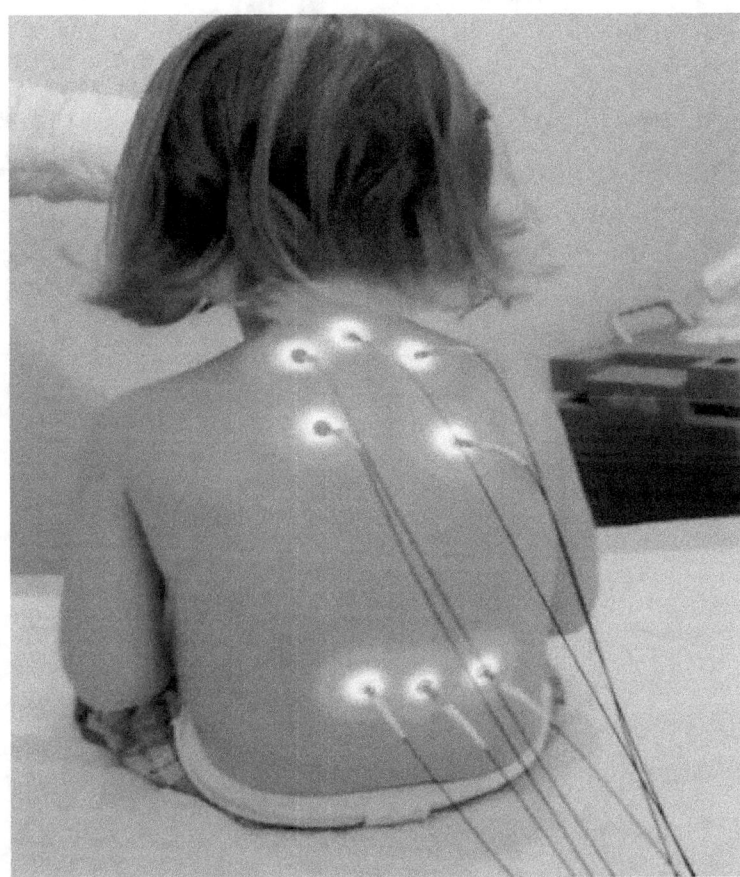

Image is sourced from www.cooperativemedicine.com/acupuncture

Editorial Note from Jan Tuner in Laser Annals
Back Issue 2. 2015

Laser acupuncture works – but how?

The results of the meta-analysis seem to be a sound scientific support for the actual existence of all the reported effects. But knowledge about the mechanisms is still scant. And ADP/ATP connection has been suggested and would make sense. But there are still many remaining questions. Is wavelength important? Which is the best energy? Does it matter?

Advancement in laser acupuncture has been seen in recent years. The "laser needle" idea makes it possible to apply high energies more precisely on the small acupuncture points. Further to that, different wavelengths can be chosen for superficial and deeply located points, and it is now possible to irradiate many acupoints at the same time, as done in needle acupuncture.

Summing up: Laser acupuncture is not placebo but similar to needle acupuncture. Enough documented to be used, especially considering the fact that it is non-invasive and pain free. Knowledge about the mechanisms will come with time. Just knowing that it is real is for the time being good enough.

SECTION SIX

ADVANCES IN SYSTEMIC TREATMENTS WITH LOW LEVEL LASER THERAPY

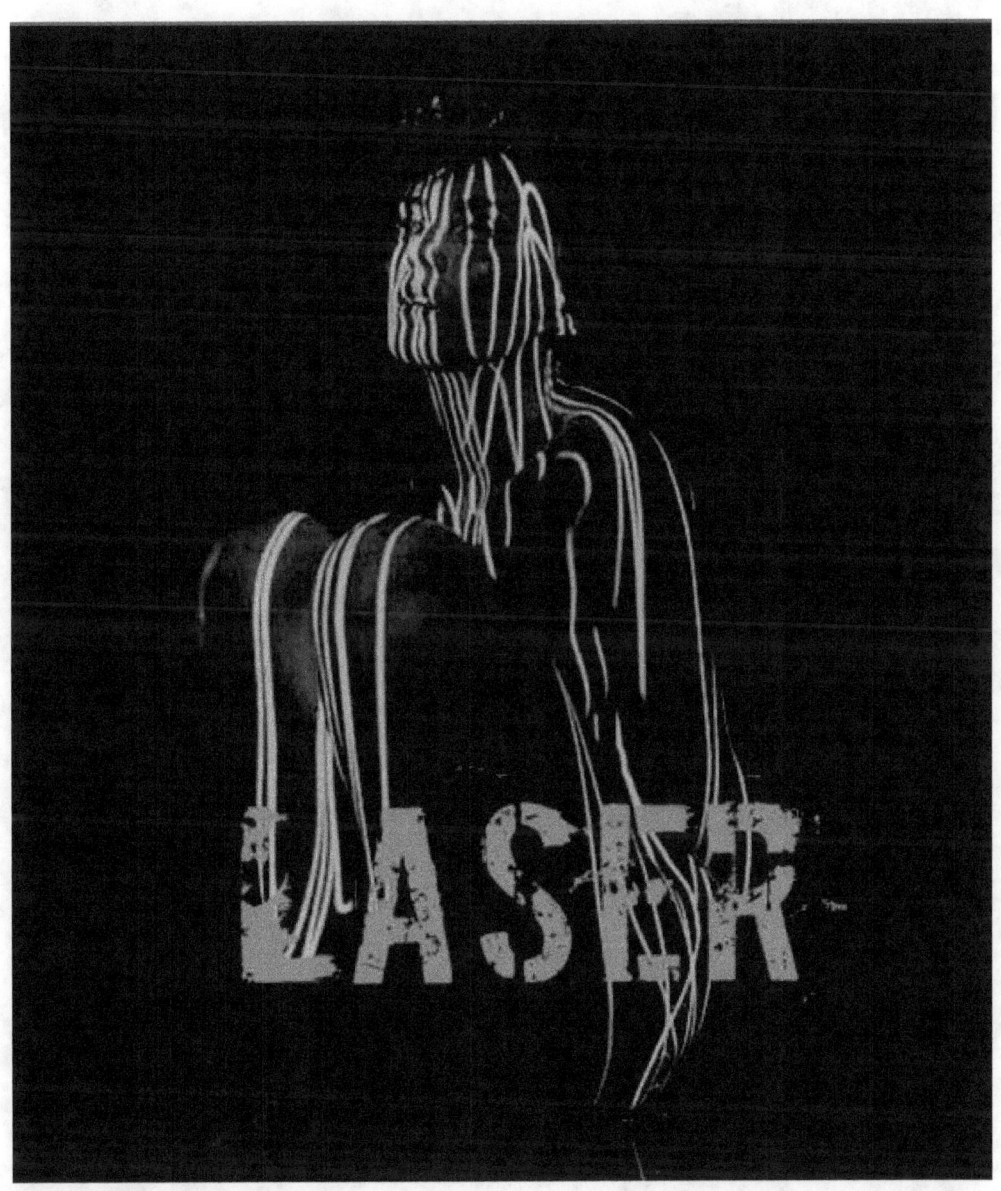

THIS IS A KNOWLEDGE SECTION BASED ON ADVANCED
TECHNICAL SKILLS IN LASER THERAPY. THE LEARNER WILL
NOT BE ASSESSED FOR KNOWLEDGE OUTCOMES INTRAVENOUS
LASER THERAPY FOR SYSTEMIC DISEASES

SKILLS DEVELOPMENT IN THIS SECTION

ADVANCED SKILLS IN BLOOD LASER THERAPY

6.1 INTRAVENOUS LOW LEVEL LASER THERAPY. ILT *(Intravenous laser therapy)*

Blood Irradiation - Introduction of a New Therapy
The method of intravenous laser blood irradiation was first introduced into therapy by the Soviet scientists E.N.Meschalkin and V.S.Sergiewski in 1981 [32].

Later Karu published significant research to contribute to the understanding of this field. Dr Michael Weber from Germany invented the Weberneedle system for popular application, and introduced a premier board dedicated to medical laser acupuncture called ISLA (International Society of Laser Acupuncture). DR Weber's system was approved by FDA, and tested by Mayo clinic with favourable outcomes.

DR Weber further introduced advances in variations of laser wavelengths used in intravenous laser, and in the combination of intravenous photosensitizers as an adjunct to intravenous laser for treatment of malignant tumours and metastases.

Effects of intravenous Low-Level-Laser-Therapy of the blood

1. Laser blood irradiation produced anti-inflammatory effects that improved the immunologic activity of the blood.

2. A fundamental finding was the positive influence on
Rheological properties of the blood which is of greatest interest to surgery, angiology and cardiology

3. A diminishing tendency of aggregation of thrombocytes and an improved deformability of erythrocytes result in an improved oxygen supply and with that to a decrease of partial which is particularly relevant to wound healing.

4. The phagocytic activity of macrophages was improved in conjunction with structural modifications.

5. A positive effect on the proliferation of lymphocytes and B- and T-cell-subpopulations could be verified too.

6. Improvement of ATP synthesis and normalization of the cell membrane potential.

7. Improved hypoxia of tissue and normalization of tissue metabolism.

8. Activation of fibrinolysis

9. Additional vasodilatation is leading to de-blocking of capillaries and collateral vessels

10. Of critical importance is the increased release of NO from monocytes with vasodilation, and improvement of endothelial dysfunction.

11. Russian surgery clinics found this method given pre operatively, could avoid post-surgery wound healing complications

12. In addition there are laser specific analgesic, spasmolytic and sedative effects. There are reports on patients with chronic glomerulonephritis who had significant improvement of tolerability of medication
(glucocorticoids, cytostatic drugs, diuretics) and of kidney function], in the same way an improvement of inflammation parameters in acute Organ pathologies has been seen along. With improved lab blood sample.

13. Formation of a larger mitochondria. This factor is used in tumour therapy to normalize gene function

14. There appears to be generalized effects of the intravenous blood-irradiation on almost every organ system so that this therapy may be employed in the treatment of various diseases causally or additively. Gasparyan described the improvement of microcirculation especially in central nervous structures. In particular, this is most important in the hypothalamus which has a highly developed vascular micro system. He assumes that the intravenous blood-irradiation is stimulating the functional activity of the hypothalamus and limbic system leading to an activation of hormonal, metabolic, immunological and vegetative processes with mobilization of adaptive reserves.

IS INTRAVENOUS LASER A 'BLOOD ACUPUNCTURE?'

In Chinese medicine Blood or 'Xue' is vital to therapy and a pervasive influence.

'Qi' or vital energy is closely linked and commands the blood. Intravenous laser may directly stimulate the blood and all its factors. Acupuncture is the stimulation of Qi with a specific outcome. Intravenous laser stimulates the Qi and moves the blood, which otherwise stagnates and deteriorates.

Science has been puzzled at the amazing curative potential that the body manifests to selfheal.

Mystics maintain that the Qi of acupuncture is the secret, untapped genetic reservoir of healing energy stored in the kidney (Chinese concept
Of kidney). Perhaps stimulating the blood energy manifests other latent self-curative potentials in the body. Perhaps blood acupuncture is another dimensional power than acupuncture from the periphery as blood pathways may act as their own internal meridian. This theory has been acceptable.

Acupuncture is a means of immortality, based on interpretation of the Classics, whereby Shen (Heart Qi associated with blood) must merge with Jing (Kidney Qi or genetic potential) in a permanent state to evolve into an everlasting life.

TREATMENT DATA IN 2005 by Weber

114 patients with a variety of clinical syndromes had been treated and evaluated in the year 2005 by Dr Weber. The treatments were carried out according to Russian instructions as combined treatments with laser needle acupuncture. Partly it concerned patients who previously showed unsatisfactory results with acupuncture exclusively.

- fat metabolism disorders (n = 20)
- diabetes mellitus (n = 20)
- chronic pain syndrome (n = 12)
- rheumatoid arthritis (n = 5)
- polyneuropathies (n = 4)
- chronic-inflammatory bowel diseases (n = 5)
- fibromyalgia (n = 7)
- hypertension (n = 6)
- tinnitus (n = 3)
- macular degeneration (n = 4)
- multiple sclerosis (n = 9)
- burn-out-syndrome (n = 9)

• allergies and eczemas (n = 10)

The following effects could be verified by a questionnaire survey and the evaluation of clinical tests and laboratory parameters:

General Effects

• significant improvement of general fitness
• improvement of sleeping behaviour and vigilance
• positive effect on general mood
• reduction of drug consumption
• optimization of diabetic metabolism
• significant lowering of pathological increased liver values
• reduction of relapse in chronic-inflammatory bowel diseases
• improvement of general well-being and mobility in multiple sclerosis
• positive influence on therapy-resistant pain syndromes
• in some cases positive influencing of tinnitus (ringing in the ear)
• reduction of antihypertensive medication in severe hypertension

Side Effects

No known side effects have appeared in the use of this therapy. Disposable catheters are now available, eliminating the need for sterilization. Laser is used in small powers as 1 – 3 mws and for 20 - 60 minutes for 10 daily sessions.

SCOPE OF APPLICATIONS

Intravenous laser has scope for providing relief to systemic diseases:

Alleries and eczemas
Diabetes
Circulatory disorders
Chronic liver and kidney diseases.
Chronic pain syndromes
Rheumatoid arthritis
Polyneuropathy
Fibromyalgia
Chronic inflammatory bowel diseases
Hypertension

Tinnitus
Multiple sclerosis
Chronic fatigue syndrome

It also has scope of treating cancer and metastases in Photodynamic therapy

Method: practical application of Intravenous Laser blood Irradiation:

Intravenous laser blood irradiation is carried out with low power of 1-3 mw and an exposure time of 20-60 minutes. A series of 10 treatments will be carried out either every day or three times a week with a weekend break.
M. H. Weber

For intravenous laser blood irradiation first of all the PT has to feed in a cannula into a suitable vein of the elbow or the forearm. The vein should have a wide lumen to catch a great volume of blood in the period of time. In the Russian studies a simple steel-cannula was inserted in which a disposal laser plastic-catheter was fed in and was connected to a laser diode. This procedure was modified by the author by feeding in a blue plastic cannula into a suitable vein and then a newly developed disposable laser-catheter made of biological compatible plastic material is inserted into the vein. With veins that are difficult to puncture or if there is lack of practice, the setting of the cannula may cause problems, but recently a suitable little butterfly was developed which permits an easy application of the above described catheter. The advantage of this therapy is that it can be learned by an assistant or a nurse, so the doctor has not to be right next.

THE GREEN INTRAVASCULAR LASER

Green laser has a shorter wavelength in the 530 nm range. It has been necessary in intravenous laser as it complements the action of the red laser. The red laser works on leucocytes and not on erythrocytes. A green laser, combined with red laser, completes all necessary actions on leucocytes and erythrocytes.

In some experiments it could be seen that the green laser had an advantage on rheologic properties of the blood by an improved deformability of erythrocytes. The corresponding absorption spectrum for haemoglobin was assumed as cause for the green laser effect in particular.

The effect of green laser light on Na-Ka-ATPase was investigated. A distinct stimulating effect of the green laser light on the activity of the erythrocyte Ka-Na-ATPase was shown. These latest findings are of exceptional significance. Previous explanatory models of the photo biochemical energy transfer model followed the mitochondrial structures and the electron carrier systems in the respiratory chain, but these are not existing in erythrocytes. According to previous ideas an absorption of green laser photons to the erythrocytes would be only transferred into a local warming up. The evidence of an increased Na-Ka-ATPase permits the conclusion that besides the warming up also structural molecular changes are activated with triggering of specific biochemical activity. So the membrane-ous lipid layers can also change.

In 2005 investigations discovered that under green light irradiation there was an increase of fibroblast proliferation with an improved effect on glucose metabolism.

THE BLUEINTRAVASCULAR LASER

The blue laser has a distinct absorption for porphyrins on account of its wavelength of 400-470 nm, so consequently for haemoglobin too . So far there are only a few scientific data of clinical application with patients since it succeeded just a short time ago to build a solid blue semiconductor laser from gallium nitride. It became public that caries, periodontosis and acne can be treated with blue LED (light-emitting diode) with good success because they are also emitting monochromatic light (but without deep-acting coherence).According to late researches Helicobacter pylori can be eradicated successfully by application of blue light over the gastro scope. Cause of these effects is the bactericide effect of the blue monochromatic light that is binding to bacterial porphyrins and destroying them by release of reactive oxygen radicals.

Tiina Karu showed in several works that in the mitochondrial respiratory chain the red as well as the infrared laser light stimulates the last complex of the respiratory chain, the so called cytochrome-C-oxidase, while the first complex, the so called NADH-dehydrogenase, has its absorption maximum in the blue range. So it is possible to stimulate this "starter complex" by irradiating with blue laser. This effect will be of considerable importance for the intravenous laser blood irradiation.

Gasparyan provided the first data. He was able to show that under irradiation of the blood with blue laser light of low power (0.3 mw) the rheology of the blood will be significantly improved and as a result the microcirculation will improve too.

According to the latest data collected by him also cases of tinnitus resistant to other therapies can be treated more successfully than before. Furthermore it was reported that metabolism effects lead to a significant decrease of cholesterol, triglycerides and blood-glucose and bilirubin. The immunologic activity of the blood is increasing significantly according to Gasparyan. Due to its proximity to the ultraviolet spectrum it is assumed that in the therapy of the blood the blue laser is also inducing the well-known immune stimulating effects as they are known from the UVB-treatment of the blood. In a work from October 2006 the blue laser was also used diagnostically to trace tumour cells.

Due to strong absorption impulses of the blue laser cause circulating melanoma-cells in the blood to swing and to emit signals that can be recorded with highly sensitive microphones.

This is called photo acoustic detection

COMPARISON OF ABSORPTION OF BLUE LASER AND RED /IR LASER:

Source: Karu: Low-Power Laser Therapy:
350 – 450 nm blue (flavoproteins, dehydrogenases)
600 – 820 nm red/infrared (cytochrome-c-oxydasis)
In the blue range (about 400 nm) the light is mainly absorbed by the NADH-dehydrogenase complex, the starter complex of the respiratory chain in the mitochondria.

In the red and infrared range between 630 and 900 nm the photons are activating mainly the complex of cytochrome-c-oxydasis, the final carrier of the respiratory chain.

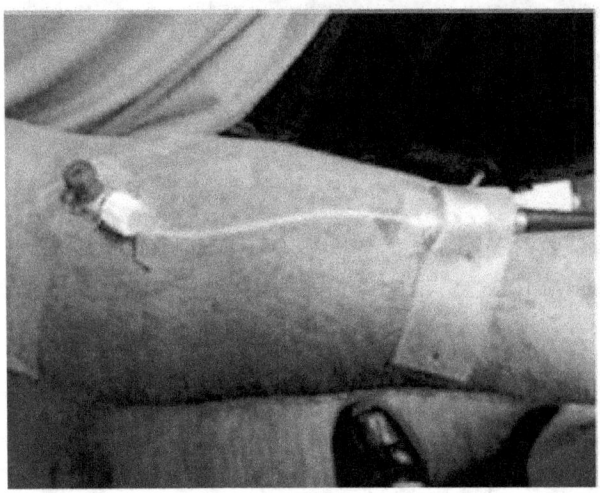

Intravenous LASER irradiation of Blue Laser. From Weber Medical

HIGHLIGHTS

THE BLUE LASER releases NO. This increases blood flow.
Blue laser is indicated for microcirculation and metabolic disorders, kidney failure and hypertension.

Green laser irradiation (532 nm) is leading to a significant increase of the sodium/potassium- ATP-ase of the erythrocytes.
Red and IR laser have deep penetration and stimulate tissue at deep level. It stimulates monocytes and macrophages, and improves immunity. It develops the giant mitochondria and increased ATP.

6.2 PHOTODYNAMIC THERAPY

Photodynamic therapy is used for the treatment of tumours and metastases.
It is a specialized therapy which employs the use of a photosensitizer prior to ILT.

Chlorophyll may be topically applied or injected locally or intravenously into the area affected by cancer. Chlorophyll absorbs far more photons inside the body, and the targeted tissue undergoes a return to normal gene expression. Tumours are noticed to dissolve. This therapy is only relevant to the Physical therapist, in order to understand advances in cancer treatment through this technology.

There should be no attempts to treat cancer with laser or led light using any systemic treatment, except with the use of an approved photosensitizer, and complete hospital care under the authority of a recognized medical practitioner.

Patients requiring treatment may be referred to a weber medical clinic for clinical therapy.

Weber needle therapy is now available on you tube with lectures from DR Weber.

Continued Profile of Jan Tuner

JAN TUNER : Continuation of reference list of his scientific published work2-Papers:

Tunér J, Hode L. It´s all in the parameters: a critical analysis of some well-known negative studies on low-level laser therapy. J Clinical Laser Med & Surgery. 1998; 16 (5): 245-248.Tunér J, Hode L. Are all the negative studies really negative? Laser Therapy. 1998; 10 (4165174.

Tunér J. 100 double-blind studies: enough or too little? Proc. SPIE. Vol. 4166 (1999). Progress in Biomedical Optics and Imaging. A Window on the Laser Medicine World. Eds Longo L. et al. P. 226-232.

Tunér J, Hode living tissue at different wavelengths, power densities and incident target areas. Proc. SPIE, Vol. 4166 (1999). Progress in Biomedical Optics and Imaging. A Window on the Laser Medicine World. Eds Longo L. et al. P.294-302.

Hode L, Tunér J. Low-level laser therapy (LLLT) versus light emitting diode therapy (LEDT); what is the difference? Proc. SPIE. Vol. 4166 (1999). Progress in Biomedical Optics and Imaging. A Window on the Laser Medicine World. Eds Longo L. et al. P. 90-97.

Tunér J. The Cochrane analyses, can they be improved? Laser Therapy. 1999; 11 (3): 138-143.

Tunér J. Lågeffektslaser – missbrukad, missförstådd. [Low level laser – misused, misunderstood]. Sjukgymnasten. 2, 2000 (The Physiotherapist, Sweden)

Tunér J. What is in the LLLT literature? In: Lasers in Medicine and Dentistry, Ed. Simunovic Z. European Medical Laser Ass. 2000, p.217-226.

Hode L, Tunér J. Depth of penetration of laser light in tissue. Laser Partner Clinixperience. 2000; (15).

Tunér J. Low Level Laser Therapy – Is There a Documentation? Laser Partner Clinixperience. 2000; (10).

Tunér J. Low level laser therapy of tinnitus - a case for the dentist? Proc. SPIE. Vol. 4422. 2000, p. 106-112.

Tunér J, Christensen P H. Low-level lasers – new possibilities in dentistry. Dental Product Reports Europe. 2000 (21) 6: 12-17.

Tunér J. Low level laser therapy. Wavelength (Academy of Laser Dentistry, USA), 2001; 9 (1): 15-16.

Tunér J. Laserterapi – myt eller möjlighet? [Laser therapy – myth or possibility?]. Nordisk Tidsskrift for Biologisk Medicin 2001; 1 (2): 20-24.

En riktig Robinson-ö. Populär Historia, October 2002. (About Dom Fernao Lopes, the first inhabitant of St Helena island – (Popular History journal).

Bjordal J M, Couppé C, Chow R T, Tunér J, Ljunggren A E. A systematic review of low level laser therapy with location-specific doses for pain from chronic joint disorders. Australian J Physiotherapy. 2003; 49: 107-116.

Tunér J, Bjorne A. What is the role of the laser dentist in the treatment of tinnitus? In: Proc. 4th Congress. WALT. MonduzziEditore, Bologna, Italy 2002.

Tunér J, Bjorne A. Somatosensory tinnitus – a case for the laser dentist. In: Lasers in Surgery, Medicine and Dentistry. Ed: Simunovic Z. Laaxus AG, Switzerland, 2003: 217-226.

Tunér J. Terapilaser inom tandvården – historik och litteratur. [Therapeutic lasers in dentistry – history and literature]. J Swed Dental Assoc. 2003; 2.

Sun G, Tunér J. Low Level Laser Therapy in Dentistry. Dental Clinics of North America. 2004: 1061-1076.

Guerra A, Munoz P, Sanchez T, Boullón J, Tunér J. The effect of 670 nm Laser Therapy on herpes simplex and aphtae. Photomedicine and Laser Surgery. 2005, 23:90. (abstract)

Qadri T, Miranda L, Tunér J, Gustafsson A. The effects of therapeutic lasers in periodontal inflammation. J Clin Periodontology. 2005; 32 (7): 714-719.

Almeida-Lopes L, Lopes A, Tunér J, Calderhead RG. Infrared diode laser therapy-induced lymphatic drainage for inflammation in the head and neck. Laser Therapy. 2005; 14 (2): 67-74.

Tunér J, Hode L. Standards for laser therapy studies. J Wound Care. 2005 Nov;14(10):478-9; author reply 478. Comment on: J Wound Care. 2005 Sep;14(8):391-4.

Hode L, Tunér J. Wrong parameters can give just any results. Lasers Surg Med. 2006; 38 (4): 343.

Qadri T, BohdaneckaP ,Tunér J, Gustafsson A. The importance of coherence length in laser phototherapy of gingival inflammation – a pilot study. Lasers in Medical Science. 2007; 22 (4) :245-251.

Bjordal JM, Tunér J, Iversen VV, Frigo L et al. A systematic review of post-operative pain relief by Low Level Laser Therapy (LLLT) after third molar extraction. Lasers in Medical Science, 2007; 22 (4): 303.

Bradley P, Tunér J. Laser Phototherapy in Dentistry. In: Proc. of the 1st Int Workshop of Evidence Based Dentistry on Lasers in Dentistry. Ed: Gutknecht N. Quintessence Books. 2007:149-171.

Laser phototherapy (LPT): expanding the scope of dentistry. Coherencia, 2009:1. Monterrey, Mexico.

Laser phototherapy in dentistry. Odontología actual. Monterrey, Mexico, 2009.

Tunér J. Is low-power pulsed laser ineffective in neural growth? Microsurgery 2009; 29 (3):251.

Qadri T, Poddani P, Javed F, Tunér J, Gustafsson A. A short-term evaluation of Nd:YAG laser as an adjunct to scaling and root planing in treatment of chronic periodontitis. J of Periodontology, 2010 Aug;81(8):1161-1166.

Qadri T, Poddani P, Javed F, Tunér J, Gustafsson A. Long–term effects of a single application of Nd:YAG laser in supplement to scaling and root planing in patients with periodontitis. Lasers in Medical Science; 2011 Nov;26(6):763-766. PMID: 20582610

Tunér J, Kristensen P H. Laser phototherapy (LPT) in dentistry. Laser Journal, International edition. Oemus Publishing, Germany, 2010.

Carlos de Paula Eduardo Patricia Moreira de Freitas, Marcella Esteves-Oliveira, Ana CecíliaCorrêaAranha, Karen Müller Ramalho, AlyneSimões, Marina Stella Bello-Silva, Jan Tunér. Laser Phototherapy in the Treatment of Periodontal Disease: A literature review. Lasers in Medical Science. 2010 Nov;25(6):781-792.

Jan Tunér, Per Hugo Kristensen. Low Level Lasers in Dentistry. In: Robert A Convissar (ed). Principles and Practice of Laser Dentistry.Pp 263-281. Mosby Elsevier Inc. 2010. ISBN 9 780323 062060.

Tunér J, Hode L. Low level laser therapy for hand arthritis – fact or fiction? ClinRhematol, 2010 Sep;29(9):1075- 1076.

Makhlouf M, Dahaba M, Eissa S, Tunér J, Harash T. A Clinical, Immunological, and Digital Radiographic Study on the Effect of Low Level Laser on Chronic Periodontitis. Dissertation; University of Cairo, Egypt, 2010.

AlyneSimões, Mariana AparecidaBrozoski, Patrícia Moreira de Freitas, Jan Tunér, Carlos de Paula Eduardo. Laser as an auxiliary therapy for Stevens Johnson Syndrome: a case report. Photomed Laser Surg. 2011 Jan;29(1):67-69.

Tunér J. Therapeutic lasers expand the scope of dentistry. BioOptics World. September 2010. p. 26-30.

Makhlouf M, Dahaba M, Eissa S, Tunér J, Harash T. A Clinical, Immunological, and Digital Radiographic Study on the Effect of Low Level Laser on Chronic Periodontitis. Photomedicine and Laser Surgery. 2012; 30 (2): 160-166.

Ramalho KM, Luiz AC, de Paula Eduardo C, Tunér J, Magalhães RP, GallottiniMagalhães M. Use of laser phototherapy on a delayed wound healing of oral mucosa previously submitted to radiotherapy: case report. Int Wound J. 2011 Aug;8(4):413-418.

Muñoz Sanchez PJ, Capote Femenías JL, DíazTejeda A, Tunér J. The effect of 670 nm low laser therapy on herpes simplex type 1. Photomedicine and Laser Surgery. 2012; 30 (1): 37-40.

Tunér J. Laser phototherapy (LPT) in dentistry. Laser – the international C.E. magazine of laser dentistry. US Edition. No 1 (1); 2011: 8-17.

Toomarian L, Fekrazad R, Tadayon N, Ramezani J, Tunér J. Stimulatory effect of low-level laser therapy on root development of rat molars: a preliminary study. Lasers Med Sci. 2012; 27 (3): 537-542.

Bjordal JM, Bensadoun RJ, Tunér J, Frigo L, Gjerde K, Lopes-Martins RA. A systematic review with metaanalysis of the effect of low-level laser therapy (LLLT) in cancer therapy-induced oral mucositis. Support Care Cancer. 2011;19(8):1069-1077.

Complications in comparing lasers and LED. Comment on Esper MA, Nicolau RA, Arisawa EA (2011) The effect of two phototherapy protocols on pain control in orthodontic procedure - a preliminary clinical study. Lasers Med Sci 26:657-663.

Qadri T, Tunér J. Some aspect of the use of Nd:YAG laser in periodontal therapy. Laser Journal, International edition. Oemus Publishing, Germany, 2012.

Muñoz Sánchez P J, Capote Femenias J L, Tunér J. Treatment of aphthous stomatitis using Low Level Laser Therapy (LLLT). Submitted 2013.

Ahrari F, Madani AS, Ghafouri ZS, Tunér J. The efficacy of low-level laser therapy for the treatment of myogenoustemporomandibular joint disorder. Lasers Med Sci. 2013 Jan 15. [Epub ahead of print]

Carlos de Paula Eduardo, Ana Cecilia CorrêaAranha, AlyneSimões, Marina Stella Bello- Silva, Karen Muller Ramalho, Marcella Esteves –Oliveira, Patríci a Moreira de Freita, Juliana Marotti, Jan Tunér. Laser Treatment of Recurrent Herpes Labialis: A Literature Review. Lasers Med Sci 2013, [Epub ahead of print]

Qadri T; Túner J; Gustafsson A .Significance of Scaling and Root Planing With Adjunctive Use of a Water-cooled Pulsed Nd:YAG Laser for the Treatment of Periodontal Inflammation. Submitted 2013.

Courses: Masters program, Instituto de Tecnología Avanzada, Monterrey, Mexico

Masters program, RWTH Aachen University, Germany

Master program, UniversitatRoviraiVirgili, Reus, Spain

Certification program of The Swedish Laser Medical Society

This manual is based on a distant education continuing professional development course.

Scientific references are not mentioned as the course is based on External verification from a technical regulating board, ISTE.

Those interested in registering for the course through virtual classes and portfolio assessment may enquire with the author at malini@bitrix24.com, or sign up at http://centerforwellness.eliademy.com

The Authors other works in Alternative medicine are available on http://amazon.com/author/malinichaudhri

www.ingramcontent.com/pod-product-compliance
Lightning Source LLC
Chambersburg PA
CBHW081724220526
45468CB00008B/1959